Assertiveness and the Manager's Job

Annie Phillips

Independent Health Advisor
Management Consultant to General Practice

Radcliffe Medical Press Ltd
18 Marcham Road
Abingdon
Oxon OX14 1AA
United Kingdom

www.radcliffe-oxford.com
The Radcliffe Medical Press electronic catalogue and online ordering facility.
Direct sales to anywhere in the world.

British Library Cataloguing in Publication Data

A catalogue record for this book is available from the British Library.

ISBN 1 85775 901 X

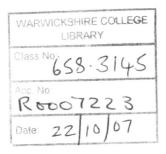

Typeset by Advance Typesetting Ltd, Oxfordshire
Printed and bound by TJ International Ltd, Padstow, Cornwall

Contents

Foreword

This book is written at a time when all managers in healthcare are taking stock of their position following the inquiries into children's cardiac surgery at the Bristol Royal Infirmary and organ retention at Alder Hey. In 1991, with the introduction of fundholding in general practice, the manager's status rose, but with its demise and the introduction of primary care groups in the late nineties, and now primary care trusts, many management roles have been taken over by doctors and nurses.

There is talk of regulation for managers to bring them in line with other health professionals, and the Institute of Healthcare Management has introduced a Code of Principles to which members sign up. Thus, it is a time of uncertainty and change for managers in all sectors of healthcare. *Assertiveness and the Manager's Job* is a publication that can be of enormous support for managers in finding a more positive way forward.

Annie Phillips recognises the inequality that many managers have often felt in working with others in their teams and stresses the importance of assertiveness. She describes in detail the components of assertiveness, what they actually mean and the influences they have in carrying out the manager's job. A thought-provoking start to the book encourages us to explore these meanings in depth and then leads us to focus specifically on the role of women and their special needs in this area. However, the book is not written exclusively for women.

Having identified the needs, the following chapters each take a critical area and systematically work through how to adjust behaviour to optimise performance and job satisfaction. One of the benefits of the way the book is written is that it is possible to select a specific topic to expand understanding and to use the exercises in the chapter to practise their application. Equally, reading through the whole book ensures that the subject has been considered in depth and from all angles, with the practical examples enhancing the text.

This book will provide managers with the opportunity to progress assertively in the changing world around them.

Brenda Sawyer MSc
Fellow of the Institute of Healthcare Management
GP Tutor, Southampton, South West Hampshire and Winchester
Management Consultant
January 2002

About the author

Annie Phillips has written professionally about health and health management since she qualified as a speech and language therapist in 1978. She has over 20 years' NHS experience in primary and secondary care as a clinician and manager.

Her 10 years as a speech and language therapist led to the research and publication of an international dysphasia/dementia screening test, presented at the 1986 British Aphasiology Conference. She has won various prizes and awards for her subsequent work, and in the 1990s she was a finalist in the *Medeconomics*' Good Management Awards, and regional winner in a national British Institute of Management competition on change management.

She worked as a practice and fund manager for a five-partner training practice in central Brighton from 1989 to 1998; from then as an independent health advisor, trainer, and management consultant to general practice.

Throughout her career she has written extensively for the therapy, GP and management press. She currently writes on contemporary management issues for a range of publications, including the *Health Service Journal*, *Community Care*, *Doctor*, *Primary Care Manager* and Croner Publications, with a focus on healthcare politics and human resource management.

As a management consultant, her interest is in organisational analysis and the development of healthy organisations, with a focus on finding ways to manage stresses and conflicts, understanding and alleviating dysfunctional communication and developing effective management strategies.

Annie can be contacted via aphillips@cwcom.net or www.anniephillips.co.uk.

Acknowledgements

Thanks to all those friends who have supported me in my own personal development, especially Hazel Underwood and Kate Downs, whom I met on one of the first assertiveness workshops back in 1984; and Jo Davies and Kathy Richardson whose friendship, support and ideas have sustained me over the years.

Thanks also to all the tutors at the David Salomon's Centre in Tunbridge Wells for introducing me to the idea of change management as a process to be learnt, and to those colleagues, too numerous to mention, whose wise counsel has challenged me to continue learning – including all those who continue to teach me as I train them.

I would like to thank all those whose work I have quoted and acknowledged in the text. I have given sources of work where possible. Should you note any queries, errors or omissions, please contact the publisher.

Finally, my very special thanks as always go to Lin and Chris, for their love and encouragement, and for gracefully giving me the time out from our family commitments to continue writing.

Introduction

What is assertiveness and can anyone learn to be assertive? These questions are often asked of me as I train health service clinicians and managers. People are anxious about assertiveness – they equate it with selfishness, aggression or a lack of humour. Others feel they are not brave, or brash, enough to learn the skills. But it is possible to learn to be assertive. With time, patience and practice anyone can learn both what assertiveness is and how to be assertive.

To be assertive is to communicate clearly, honestly and directly, without avoidance or resorting to manipulative or aggressive behaviour. Part One of this book describes what assertiveness is and teaches the reader some of the skills needed to become assertive. Readers will learn here how to deal with making and refusing requests, how to deal with anger, conflict and criticism, and how to negotiate well. In Part Two you will learn how to apply some of these learned skills to common work situations – managing people, goal setting, managing change. You will also learn how to use assertiveness to manage your own time and stress levels more effectively.

Assertive people take control of situations. People who are successful do not leave anything to chance. They do not avoid conflict or difficulties or ignore problems. They take charge and confront inefficiency, unfairness, mediocrity or poor conduct with honesty and clarity, without which they could not achieve in life or work. Assertive people face their insecurities, and learn how to cope with authority. They allow themselves to make mistakes, knowing that assurance comes with experience. They know there is no such thing as the perfect boss, remembering that good intentions are as important as any other quality.

Assertive people achieve success as they bring themselves into the best possible focus. They take responsibility for using all their capabilities. They listen, ask questions, take advice and then act.

As we behave assertively we experience very positive, empowering feelings, and these feelings inevitably become more central to our lives. The new inner strength brings with it influence, authority and increased power to be used respectfully and wisely, with room allowed for negotiation. In learning to be assertive you begin to understand yourself, and others, more. Through being assertive you also empower others, allowing them the space to negotiate their needs.

This book will assist both the new and experienced primary care manager or clinician to become a more assertive, effective (and human!) employer or employee. Take time to read it, enjoy, and allow yourself the space to change.

Annie Phillips
January 2002

PART ONE

CHAPTER 1

The importance of being assertive

Learning to be assertive has become a popular form of self-development; it is seen as an important component in cognitive-behavioural approaches to tackling anger, anxiety, depression, and poor self-esteem. The premise is that changing people's ideas influences their behaviour; likewise changing behaviour leads to changes in ideas.[1–3]

Assertive techniques help us to communicate in constructive and satisfying ways, achieve workable results in difficult situations and can assist in resolving conflicts without aggression. They are essential techniques to understand and use as managers, particularly for health and social care managers, who juggle with their roles as clinician, carer, manager, support worker, facilitator, etc. We draw constantly on our emotional and intellectual resources when dealing with practice conflicts and we struggle to provide a good service with limited resources and little peer group support. We can also feel very guilty when we don't, or are unable to, live up to the caring image. If we identify with the image that we do not want to let others down, we can easily absorb others' concerns and worries as we do not want to be a disappointment to people or be seen to be selfish. We often like to be thought of as indispensable – our work can involve sacrifice, we find it hard to delegate and certainly do not want to offend.

Some facts about assertiveness

- To be assertive is not to behave selfishly.
- The assertive person recognises their own limits and is able to call things to a halt before they burn out.
- They give themselves time to rest and replenish their energies.
- They recognise their needs are no more or no less than others, but equal.

Some of the situations that assertive behaviour can help with:

- time management
- identification of obstacles to career or personal development
- relaxation
- overcoming work, people and time demands
- making and refusing requests
- handling criticism or compliments
- coping with rejection
- building self-esteem
- giving constructive criticism
- staff appraisals and disciplinary procedures
- negotiating
- dealing effectively with conflict and violence
- goal setting.

Behaving assertively helps at both a professional and personal level. It helps us to communicate directly and powerfully at work, and can also defend against aggression or defensive behaviour when hopes and plans are thwarted. Negotiation and compromise form the lynch pin in assertiveness training. The assertive person takes charge and acts in ways that invite respect, accepting their own limitations and strengths. This in turn leads to clearer communication, as others understand clearly what their needs and desires are, and any potential confusion or discord is alleviated.

Practice managers are unique in their role as representatives of general practice: they act as advocates for the staff and patients; they lead and yet are in turn 'managed' by their employers, the GPs. These unusual relationships can cause conflict. Assertive skills enable us to see our role more clearly and cope more readily with feelings of frustration or inadequacy. We need to be able to express anger and anxiety clearly in order to prevent further stress.

Anne Dickson, an American psychologist, wrote one of the first books on assertiveness.[4] Dickson's excellent work is the source of much of the material subsequently written on assertiveness in this country. She promoted assertiveness training as a popular method for gaining greater self-confidence and control over one's life, but also warned that it does not mean:

- *you will always get what you want*. Other people may be indifferent or hostile to your declaration of rights
- *you must always be assertive*. Assertiveness is one option among many others – be prudent or selective
- *people will always respect or like you*. Your relationships may change as you do
- *being assertive equals strength*. Choose when to be assertive
- *you are a good person*. Basing self-worth on a particular behaviour can quickly lead to self-depreciation
- *all of your problems will be solved.* Assertiveness is one tool among many.

Do you see yourself as:

Passive?

- You are tearful, frustrated.
- You are a victim.
- You opt out of making decisions.
- Others try to help, but this is never enough.
- You are negative, resigned, whining.
- You self-negate and self-pity.
- You internalise stress.

Aggressive?

- You are angry, defensive, competitive.
- You put others down.
- You have low self-esteem, and often confront and attack.
- You over-react, others feel hurt, humiliated and resentful.
- You release anger at the expense of others.

Manipulative?

- You get your own way through flirting, pandering to egos.
- You have low self-esteem.
- You are indirect, subtle.
- You fear exposure, it is safer to control and manipulate than risk rejection.
- You are devious.
- You meet any attempt to clarify with denial.

Assertiveness is:

- saying what you want without resorting to anger or manipulation
- respecting people
- accepting our own positive and negative feelings
- more tolerant, less judgemental
- taking responsibility for ourselves
- acknowledging our own needs
- asking directly
- risking refusal
- having good self-esteem
- not being dependent on others
- setting limits and boundaries.

There are said to be four *ego states*:[5]

FREE CHILD	ADULT
ADAPTIVE CHILD	CRITICAL PARENT

And four ways of interacting:

I'm ok –	you're ok	(adult)
I'm ok –	you're not ok	(the bully)
I'm not ok –	you're not ok	(the aggressive victim)
I'm not ok –	you're ok	(depressed)

The assertive person would respond as an adult, neutrally and fairly. How would you respond?

> 'I'd like to ask a favour. Since you're going to be away for a week, I'm wondering if I could borrow your car? Our second car is out of action and my wife needs one to take the kids to school.' Your reply:
>
> Passive
>
> Aggressive
>
> Assertive

All of us have the right to be treated with respect, to be listened to and taken seriously. We have the right to set our own priorities and choose for ourselves. We have the right to express our own feelings and opinions – including saying no – without fear. We have the right to make mistakes.

It is especially important for primary care workers to use assertiveness skills as we care for the patients, staff, and for the health service. We therefore can feel very guilty when we don't, or are unable to, live up to the caring image. We often like to be thought of as indispensable; our work can involve sacrifice and we often find it hard to delegate. We do not want to offend and so it is extremely easy for us to feel guilty. Consider the following scenarios.

- You feel guilty about taking any time out – you need to be available to your practice at all times.

- You do not move to a more stimulating or rewarding job because you know your practice will have difficulty replacing you.
- You do not push the partners as hard as you should because you can empathise with their difficulties of increasing patient demands.
- You do not ask your staff not to smoke in a no smoking area because you sympathise with their need to smoke under pressure.
- You reluctantly accept a new system of working that you have reservations about because you don't want to offend the partner who is enthusiastic about it.

Anyone who consistently behaves in this way will quickly over-stretch and exhaust themselves. They are taking care of everyone else but themsleves, at a huge cost to their own physical and mental well-being. They think of themselves as inexhaustible, but will soon 'burn out'.

The compassion trap

Using the columns below, list those things that you do for other people because they ask you, not because you want to do them.

Work	Friendships	Home

For example:

Work	Friendships	Home
Always make the coffee Stay late on Fridays Take on call every Christmas	Always lend my car	Housework Go to parent's evening

Then swap lists with a friend, and try role-playing, saying 'no' politely but firmly. If you feel you need more practice, *see* Chapter 5, Making and refusing requests.

How to change

To be assertive is not to behave selfishly. The assertive person recognises their own limits and is able to call things to a halt before they burn out. They give themselves time to rest and replenish their energies, so that when they do give once more they do so with strength and enthusiasm.

Do you:

- find delegation difficult
- assume responsibility for other people's needs
- deny people equal rights of interaction
- organise other people's lives
- make decisions for friends, family and co-workers
- assume that people cannot manage by themselves.

Here you are taking inappropriate responsibility for other people's lives. Women, in particular, are reluctant to relinquish this power, as it is perhaps the only area of their life where they hold it. If this is the case, by taking more power for yourself assertively you will feel able to give up this strong manipulative hold and claim real equality.

You will still be able to show compassion, love and care to others, but the choice will be yours and you will not be compelled to always put others' needs before your own.

Your rights

We all have needs, rights, opinions and choices but because of cultural pressures, those in less powerful positions can find it difficult acknowledging that they are entitled to these, the paradox is that they understand, acknowledge and fulfil other people's all the time! When we acknowledge that we too have certain rights, we set ourselves free from the dependence on others for their approval.

- We fear disapproval because it threatens our sense of self.
- We may have felt hurt and unloved when younger.
- This fear (of losing love) can then easily shift to other respected, or authority figures in our lives – especially those at work.
- We want to be liked, so in anticipating disapproval we avoid stating our needs.

Consider the following example.

Hazel is a successful and respected practice manager. She pioneered a surgery move and the development of some new, innovative patient services. She has acted as the catalyst for a lot of positive change. She has decided, after much consideration, that she wishes to resign and move on, after only 18 months in post.

Her employers plead with her. They ask her why she is leaving; they are concerned that the practice will collapse without her. Hazel feels caught in a trap. She feels the need of her staff and the partners and is concerned that she will appear selfish if she leaves so soon. Maybe she should carry on for another few years. She feels guilt and sympathy for her colleagues left to manage by themselves. Eventually she states her position assertively. She acknowledges the partner's position and explains that she feels that a lot of her time and energy has been given to this particular job. Although she has enjoyed the job tremendously, it would be fairer, and also healthier, for someone else to have a chance. The others hear her and respect her clarity and decision; she herself leaves feeling satisfied that she has made the right choice.

Hazel was allowing herself to have needs. She needed time, a change of scene, and a different challenge. Had she stayed in post she would have become stale and possibly resentful. The explanation she gave to her colleagues demonstrated her concern for the practice, but also showed them that she too had needs and other plans that she wished to fulfil. She chose for herself assertively.

Anne Dickson sets out what has come to be known as *A Bill of Rights*, pin it up somewhere.[4]

I have the right to:

Be treated with respect

Set my own priorities

Ask for what I want

Be listened to and taken seriously

Set my own goals

Say 'no' without feeling guilty

Express my own feelings and opinions

Make mistakes

Ask for, and obtain information from professionals

Receive criticism in my own way

Get what I pay for

Choose for myself

These rights are examined overleaf in more detail. What do they mean for us in primary care?

I have the right to be treated with respect

In a system where both doctors and medical managers regard power inequalities as natural, necessary and beneficial, this is hard. Doctors tend to attach little value to having a supportive superior, and back a medical ascendancy model of management. The present culture may work for medics, but it certainly does not work for the co-workers. Within this system:

- it is very difficult for a non-doctor to have and offer opinions
- it is very easy to forget that what we feel and what we have to say as an intelligent and informed individual does count
- there is always someone ready and willing to put you in your place.

We need to remember in these circumstances that our own needs and opinions matter too. Being treated with respect means:

- being noticed – there are many occasions when a manager's opinions are not sought; they are ignored
- others may not agree with what you have to say but at least you have a right to a voice
- that your time is valued and appreciated, e.g. people cannot always assume that they can talk with you at their own convenience.

I have the right to set my own priorities

If you are feeling disempowered it is very easy to let others lead your agenda. Set your own priorities. One of these might be the need to set aside time for yourself so you can see yourself as someone who deserves as much time, effort and energy as your family, the practice and the patients. If you permit yourself the right to look after your own life, the need for others to speak for you is removed. Once you give yourself silent permission to set your own priorities the balance of power is redressed if someone pressures you to follow their agenda. Let us take an example.

> Kate is a practice manager who has allocated some time in her day to review the practice accounts. The practice is busy dealing with a flu epidemic, but among other pressures and deadlines, Kate has to review these accounts prior to a meeting with the accountant the following day. She wants to present a summary to the senior partner at their lunchtime review. When she arrives in her office, one of the partners rushes in to greet her in a panic. He asks her if she could possibly cover reception, as they are short-staffed and it is a Monday morning. Kate acknowledges the partner's difficulties, but reasserts her need and wish to continue with the work she is doing. She will, however, do her utmost to obtain locum cover, and picks up the phone instantly to set this in motion. Kate,

as a fellow professional, has set her own limits and priorities for the day. She does not need to allow the senior partner to organise her, as she is capable of organising herself.

I have the right to ask for what I want

Here you establish your right to identify and communicate your needs as an equal. It is easy, especially when you are newly qualified, or new to an organisation, to feel that you do not matter, and to be in awe of others who seem much older and more experienced. All of us need to remember that we too have the right to ask for what we want, and to ask for information or clarification if we do not understand.

- Allow yourself to communicate your needs to others, remembering of course that you cannot always expect those needs to be met – allow yourself room for negotiation.
- Never accept substandard accommodation to work in. Everyone working in the public sector is entitled to accommodation that is quiet, free from distractions, and suitably furnished. Refuse to work in unsuitable premises; it is only by doing this that some respect will eventually be shown to you and your profession.
- Never allow yourself to accept rude, aggressive or undermining behaviour.
- If you do not voice your concerns your work will be undervalued.
- Ask for what you want, you have nothing to lose. If you do not ask, others will not know.

I have the right to be listened to and taken seriously

What you say may not, of course, always be right, but you do have a right to air your opinions. Do not allow your age or (apparent) lack of professional standing to belittle you. What you have to say is important to you otherwise you would not be saying it, whether you are acting in a professional capacity or not. You also have the right to make statements that may have no logical basis, without justification.

I have the right to set my own goals

- Make your own choices when decisions need to be made.
- Do not allow others to automatically choose for you.
- Set your own goals, your own standards and limits.
- Ask for that help if you need it.

It is very easy to fall into the trap of giving others the power to make our decisions for us. When we were children we looked to our parents to make important decisions on our behalf – our education, often our choice of career was a parental choice and not entirely our own. Once you are an adult, give yourself the luxury of choosing for yourself; you are capable of planning and controlling your own life.

I have the right to say no without feeling guilty

If you consistently put others' needs before your own you fall into the compassion trap mentioned previously. Allow yourself to balance out your own needs with those of other people's. Make your own decisions and choices, which include saying 'no' periodically to demands made on you. If you are being asked to do something that you feel unable or unwilling to do, think again before automatically agreeing.

I have the right to express my own feelings and opinions

- You have the right to hold an opinion, have feelings and emotions about issues, and to express them appropriately.
- Do not allow others to manipulate you or try and make you change your mind.
- Do not allow others to deny you your feelings.
- Be ready to stand by your own opinions when others try to belittle you.

The passive person would automatically concede and agree with another opinion to preserve the peace. An aggressive person would present their opinions dogmatically, denying others the right to share theirs. The assertive person respects another's opinions and feelings, while acknowledging that they hold a (possibly) differing view.

I have the right to make mistakes

Mistakes are acceptable – everyone makes them. The world does not collapse when we make one wrong move. You need to acknowledge the mistake and start afresh. In this way your self-esteem and confidence in yourself is retained. You also have the right to change your mind; this is part of taking responsibility for your own decisions and coping with the consequences.

I have the right to ask for and get information from professionals

Remember your individual, or consumer rights, when faced with professionals who often withhold information to retain power or authority.

- Do not be afraid to admit that you do not understand.
- Often an acknowledgement of your own weaknesses will be met with sympathy and respect.

- Admit to ignorance or confusion.
- Admit to not knowing.
- Ask for clarification, or for more information.
- Ask clearly and confidently, avoiding subtleties and suggestions.
- A clear, direct question should be met with an equally clear, respectful response.

I have the right to receive criticism in my own way

Allow yourself the right to accept criticism if you feel that it is fair, but ask for clarification or an example if you feel the criticism is unjustified. In this way you need not be totally demolished by personal comments or criticisms. You need not take unjustified criticism on board.

I have the right to get what I pay for

You have a right not only to return goods that are faulty, but to reflect that you deserve fair treatment from people whose services you have requested. If you attend a course that you feel was poor value for money – say so! If your boss promises to set aside an hour to discuss a problem and then takes phone calls through the discussion – air your grievance! If an informal 'contract' has been set up between two people, it is unfair for one not to keep to their side of the agreement. You deserve better treatment.

I have the right to choose for myself

The assertive person successfully assesses their own behaviour and thus releases themselves from dependence on the opinions of others.

- You have the right to choose whether or not to get involved with someone.
- You have the right to choose privacy.
- You have the right to be alone and independent.
- You have the right to be assertive.

On the left hand column of the grid below, list your own needs, the favourite things you like to do: e.g. 'I like chocolate cake', 'I like living alone'. On the right, list those people who impose on those activities and say why you can't do them.

I like eating lunch alone	Dr C wants me to eat with the staff

You can also choose when, where, and if you wish to be assertive, do not berate yourself if you cannot, or choose not, to do so.

Some blocks to assertiveness

What prevents people from being assertive?

- Fear of rejection.
- Fear of hurting others.
- Fear of violence.
- Fear of financial insecurity.
- Fear of failure.
- Lack of role models.
- Lack of opportunity to acquire skills.
- Cultural, philosophical or religious beliefs.
- Previous negative experiences.
- Anxiety.
- Procrastination.

If you have actual or emotional blocks such as those above, try and question these, and imagine the real consequences of behaving assertively.

Further help

If any of these scenarios sound familiar you need someone to be on your side. The British Association for Counselling and Psychotherapy (BACP) (tel: 01788 550899) have the names of local counsellors who can help you move on.

For more details on assertiveness courses contact The Industrial Society (tel: 0870 400 1000), your local further education college, or the author on www.anniephillips.co.uk.

References

1   Grieger R and Boyd J (1980) *Rational-Emotive Therapy: a skills based approach.* Van Nostrand Reinhold, New York, p. 187.

2   Ellis A (1979) (Audio cassette) *RETR and Assertiveness Training.* Albert Ellis Institute for Rational-Emotive Behaviour Therapy, New York.

3   Beck AT, Rush AJ, Shaw BF and Emery G (1979) *Cognitive Therapy of Depression.* Guilford, New York.

4   Dickson A (1982) *A Woman in Your Own Right.* Quartet Books, London.

5   Berne E (1968) *Games People Play.* Penguin Books, London.

Further reading

Gutmann J (1993) *The Assertiveness Workbook: a plan for busy women*. Sheldon Press, London.

Lindenfield G (2000) *Super Confidence* (2e). HarperCollins, London.

CHAPTER 2

Women at work

In this chapter we address some of the reasons why women, in particular, need to develop assertiveness skills. In this, and the following chapters, it will become apparent why men, for various physiological, psychological and sociocultural reasons, find it easier to assert themselves and carve out a place for themselves in the workplace. Many men do, of course, also need to learn to adapt their behaviour – particularly non-functional aggressive behaviour – but here we will focus on women's needs.

Consider the following.

- You go on holiday, but feel panicked by the amount of work left behind, so you phone in or return a day earlier to sort things out.
- You do not tell a doctor that he has made a mistake because it might impact badly; you find it difficult being a female managing men.
- You refuse offers of help because you feel you should be able to cope, or that you are the only one with the skills to do it properly anyway.

If you are a woman, and can identify with any of these, you are someone who denies her own needs and wishes at the expense of others. Women are brought up to have a sense of obligation to others. We make ourselves available to others to our own detriment, and, ultimately, other's too. Our compassion traps us, which is why it is important to harness some assertiveness skills.

We all have needs, rights, opinions and choices that we have a right to exercise. Because of cultural pressures, women, in particular, find it difficult to acknowledge these needs and rights and own them.

Non-assertive people:

- spend a considerable amount of time understanding, acknowledging and fulfilling other people's needs
- fear disapproval because it threatens their sense of self-esteem
- want to be liked, so avoid standing up for themselves.

Assertive people:

- successfully assess their own behaviour
- release themselves from dependence on the opinions of others
- accept their own vulnerabilities and inherent desire to be liked
- choose for themselves, freeing themselves from manipulative behaviour and resentments.

Many men have only known women as subordinates. No matter how know-ledgeable and skilled, female managers may still be perceived as flirtatious, competitive, soft or too hard. Many men feel a loss of identity, invaded, insecure and threatened by competent women. Women can assist by continuous deter-mination for a professional relationship – mutual help, information sharing and socialisation. As women model good management behaviour, they break down the prejudices and help men to form new expectations of them.

Women's advantage is their well developed communication skills. They are:

- more able at developing and maintaining communication links
- capable of building reciprocal relationships of great potential and mutual benefit
- very good at process observation
- trained to pick up other people's discomforts, anxieties, fears and angers
- able to respond to emotions instinctively.

Because of this:

- women often say much more about the way they are feeling than they feel comfortable with
- men need to be educated to become better 'process' observers
- men fail to perceive emotional cues and need to learn to respond with understanding in the same way.

We need to remember that women are also intelligent, capable and equal human beings, especially when they feel undermined by our imperialist medical system that assumes medics, and men in particular, hold the power. The health service is a hierarchical organisation with unwritten rules at play; the medics dominate the hierarchy which leaves managers in a much less powerful position. If in your workplace:

- information is withheld: only certain people are allowed access to the medical notes/information/meetings
- doctors only are permitted to prescribe, judge, decide, diagnose
- the doctors are cynical, disenchanted, defensive and obstructive of change
- medicine is still practised in an anachronistic, parochial and patriarchal way
- managers have to fight their way through the system to be heard

the balance of power is held with the medics. However, this is shifting, with those in less powerful positions gaining more confidence and authority to question the medical accendancy model. People become more assertive as they become more informed. They demand information, value for money, and are not so easily placated.

Women managers therefore need to grow into the skills demanded of them, develop their confidence and become more assertive. The first step is for women to build their self-esteem, believe in their own abilities and reduce self-blame.

Work blocks for women[1]

- *The honesty block*: you are less guarded than you need to be. Revealing only what you want to reveal is not only necessary for self-protection, but also implies the ability to keep confidences.
- *The rules block*: you take apparent rules literally. Men learn early in life that there are really two sets of rules – overt and covert.
- *The efficiency block*: you think that efficiency is key. This might be the ideal, but in business work gets done through an intricate set of relationships and office politics.
- *The niceness block*: remember you are liked or disliked on the basis of all your actions and your whole character.
- *The authority block*: you see yourself as weak, and those in authority as powerful. This prevents you from having the kind of productive team relationships with higher level people which are essential to moving ahead.
- *The political block*: the higher one goes in the workplace, the more one's success depends on being able to combine competence with political ability, a sense of strategy and human relations skills.
- *The socialisation block*: you see the social side of work as wasting time, but it may well be an essential aspect of the job once you are higher up.
- *The competition block*: you feel inadequate, and steer away from competition for fear that you will lose. Or conversely you fear you will win, and thus humiliate your competitors. However, as you develop your skills and recognise the value of competition you will fear failure less.
- *The feminine block*: you feel compelled to play a 'feminine' naïve role, and express shock and disbelief at some of the ways of the business world. This attitude doesn't win respect, but cuts you off from sources of information.

Self-blame

If you always reproach yourself when things go wrong, especially when the fault is not yours, you need to put the blame where it belongs.

If we grow up with over-critical caregivers, we realise we've broken the regulations only when we get punished.[2] As a result we develop a sensitive spot, an alarm that signals we're at fault: a sense of responsibility that is usefully triggered when we genuinely make mistakes. Less usefully, this alarm also goes off as an advance warning when a mistake has been made and it's not clear whose error it is. In response to that guilty inner flinch we quickly respond to off-load the discomfort by blaming someone else, or take the blame ourselves.

Research shows that while men look outside themselves to see why things have gone wrong, women look inside, and blame themselves. Accepting fault feels more comfortable. It:

- avoids conflict
- nurtures others
- smooths over relationships.

This can be challenged by acting in a positive and constructive way: register that in some way you could have done better and that you'll take better action next time. Taking the blame means buying into the belief that all errors are your fault. The hopelessness and negativity are destructive and do nothing to help you deal with the problem.

Accept responsibility, not blame

- Spot the physical warning signs: your stomach churning, or a voice in your head saying, 'It's my fault again'.
- Note your automatic apology and offer to put things right.
- Assess whether this is an appropriate response.
- If no, stop, reflect and start to break the pattern.

Challenge your accusers

When someone blames you what they're actually doing is off-loading their own discomfort. Men and children, in particular, will routinely shift responsibility to external circumstances – and that means you. So 'Where's my shirt?' becomes 'Where did you put my shirt?': the implication is clear.

Don't live by others' standards

Blame often arises because there is a disagreement about the right way to do things. Whatever the outcome, if you act in a way other people don't agree with, they do not approve of you. Ask yourself if you have acted in a way that meets your own standards, available energy and resources. If not, agree, and decide to act differently next time. But if you have, you have done your best; what other people feel about it is their problem.

Choose when to apologise

As a way of life, making repeated apologies is a bad idea. It:

- undermines self-confidence
- makes you feel at fault
- gives others the impression that you deserve the blame.

Instead:

- bite back the word
- replace it with 'How can I help you put that right?' or 'What's the best thing to do here?'.

Don't expect to be perfect

With expectations of women being higher than ever, blame often centres not so much on what you've done as what you haven't done. But the reality is that you can't keep a perfect house, hold down a perfect job, and be a perfect mother.

- Force yourself to lower your sights.
- Set yourself realistic standards.
- If you are running out of time, do whatever you can.
- Enlist the help of others without giving in to feelings of guilt.

Build your self-esteem

You are more likely to take the blame if you lack belief in yourself: this will be easier if you've had little experience of being good, successful or valid in life. However, if you do manage to raise your self-esteem, you will not only be able to resist your self-blaming inner voice, but you will also feel more confident to challenge others who are trying to place the blame on you.

- Learn how to be assertive, and say no.

Quick ways to reduce the blame

- Wait: listen to the other person (or the self-blame you're putting on yourself) rather than rushing in, without thinking, to apologise or explain.
- Relax: feeling physically better will make you emotionally more resilient.
- Check the messages you are sending out. Stand relaxed and easy and keep eye contact rather than looking away defensively.

Convert blame into action

- Sort out the problem that created the blame in the first place.
- Focus on what positive action you can take.
- Say to the other person or yourself: 'This is no one's fault – so how shall we sort this out?'.

The unwritten work rules

Women are expected by society to be more compliant than challenging and more obedient than ambitious. Other qualities, like leadership, taking full responsibility for the outcome of things and risk taking, are not encouraged, but these are the very things required of us in the business world.

To combat some basic stereotyping:[1]

Stereotype A: women are too interested in personal life

- Demonstrate your commitment. Women tend to be regarded as temporary members of the work force until they prove otherwise. Talk to those above you about your plans and ambitions.
- Make it a practice, *on important occasions*, to arrive early and stay late. Make it clear you do have an outside life – but you want to do what is needed because you are involved in your job.
- Let it be known that you carry business home: 'I was reading an article last night on such-and-such that suggested a solution to ...'.

Stereotype B: women are girls

- Look like a woman who takes complete financial responsibility for herself. Your career is a permanent part of your life.
- Leave your personal life at home. If you have children, make your calls to the childminder short and in break time, and don't discuss the situation with your colleagues.
- When personal problems get in the way of your work, demonstrate your reliability. Be seen as a self-sufficient adult who can handle responsibility and act on her own initiative.
- Don't just present problems: confront and solve them.
- Use the active voice. You are not asking permission. Instead of 'May I?' and 'Can I?' use 'I'm planning to' and 'I've decided to'.
- Don't appear to avoid adult responsibility by deferring to a 'parent': 'I have to ask my partner' or 'I don't know if the doctors will let me'. Put yourself in an adult role by getting your own information, and be your own decision maker.

- Do not diminish yourself: use your full adult name at work: Deborah not Debs.
- Search out role models whom you particularly admire and learn what there is about their behaviour and appearance that could help enhance your image.

Stereotype C: women aren't tough enough

The big danger for a lot of women lies in seeming too malleable. Don't think you are making an assertion just by making a protest. In negotiations, people will push hard to get the best deal they can, so if you raise an issue, make it effectual. If you postpone the issue you display weakness and compliance. Don't assume that if you are reasonable, your adversary will respond by also being reasonable. Be assertive as shown in the example below.

Asserter: 'We agreed on £3000; I simply won't pay more.'
Overcharger: 'You didn't tell us about all the difficulties. We lost hundreds of pounds.'
Asserter: 'I'm sorry you lost money, but the agreed price is £3000.'
Overcharger: 'You're being unreasonable. Everyone knows things have to be adjusted when there are problems.'
Asserter: 'I am sympathetic to your situations, but a deal's a deal.'

See Appendix A for some of the self-help exercises you can do to assist in your development:

- change some of your unwanted labels
- improve self-awareness
- identify your needs
- project your importance.

Different people have different numbers of labels. A few only have labels they like or don't like about themselves. Where do you think your labels have come from? The early years of life? More recent experiences? We may take on these labels because we feel too powerless to reject them. However, it is possible to reconsider these labels and to change them if you want to.

Labels have advantages in that they make us feel secure and comfortable, they guide our behaviour ('I am someone who always takes risks') and they give us permission to do things ('I am weak willed so I am more likely to eat extra cream'). But labels can also be dangerous, as they can keep us in fixed patterns of behaviour ('I am unemotional and never express my anger') when it is justified, and it might be better, to reveal our feelings, and they help us avoid new experiences.

Body language

Assertive messages can be conveyed verbally and non-verbally, and part of being assertive is knowing how to conduct yourself confidently using the appropriate posture, gesture and facial expressions.

This is not a question of acting. You need to *feel* assertive, not just behave as though you are, otherwise a covert message leaks out. It is difficult to disguise powerful emotions as body language reveals true feelings. It is possible, though, to build your confidence and self-esteem by simply adjusting your posture or appearance. Think how much easier it is to confront an issue if you stand face to face with someone, rather than you sitting and them standing.

See Appendix B for some ways to improve your understanding of non-verbal behaviour, e.g.:

• eye contact
• seating positions
• loudness of voice
• tone of voice
• facial expression
• body posture.

Think about the ways we behave when we are disgusted, angry or puzzled. How does it show? How do men and women differ in their non-verbal behaviour – their use of space, tone of voice?

In our (still patriarchal) society, women and children are already in a subservient space – this can be corrected by taking up as much space as men. Watch how people behave in public spaces – men confident of their position and power open their bodies up, they may sprawl their legs, arms behind their head, akimbo. They may place their possessions (briefcase, etc.) in an extended space beside them to increase their territorial range. Their voices are stronger and carry further (listen to the mobile phone users). Women do not permit themselves this privilege; their clothing is often restrictive, forcing the body to close in, restricting the space taken up and limiting the power base. We may not feel comfortable adopting men's dress or postures – who is to say these ways of behaving are sound – but we can redress the balance by taking equal space ourselves, in our own way.

Posture and distance

For assertive behaviour:

• stand or sit upright and relaxed, with your feet firmly on the ground
• deepen your breathing and calm yourself

- check to see if you are too near to the other person, which can be construed as confrontational
- whoever sits or stands in a higher position is the dominant one – raise or lower your chair to meet the other as an equal
- be still, and use open hand movements
- avoid a timid, tentative walk. Enter a room as if you belong there
- don't smile too much. Don't smile at all if it is not in keeping with the seriousness of what you are saying.

Watch out for:

- impatience, indicated through striding, leaning over or finger pointing
- dominant or aggressive behaviour: use of too much space, crossing arms to indicate inapproachability or protection
- nervous twiddling, clasping and unclasping of the hands or shuffling feet
- tapping or chopping hand movements are construed to be aggressive and impatient.

Facial expressions and intonation

Our voice is very important to us in many ways. What happens to your voice when you speak with someone on the telephone; what can you tell about them from their voice? What happens when you feel pleased and happy to see someone, or you are angry? Think of someone whose voice is easy to listen to. What qualities does the voice have?

Which of the following traits are preferable to listen to:

loud/soft	fast rate/slow	clear/imprecise enunciation
high/low pitch	tuneful/monotonous	

Thinking of these traits, try reading a passage and altering your voice. How do you sound?

The following voice features are very much interlinked:

Slow speech = more precise speech

Raised pitch = louder voice

If you relax and breathe deeply, using diaphragmatic not chest breathing, your voice will be clearer and resonate well.

For assertive behaviour

- maintain eye contact by looking at the other in a relaxed, friendly, confident way
- keep your voice steady and fluent
- speak not too loudly nor too softly
- lower your voice.

Avoid:

- covering your mouth with your hand
- smiling inappropriately – women often smile involuntarily when angry or critical (as we have been socialised to deal with angry feelings indirectly and do not feel comfortable conveying them clearly)
- whining, shouting or conveying sarcasm through the tone of your voice
- aggressive speech – clipped, fast and abrupt
- speaking over-softly, quietly or trailing off – the passive person speaks quietly and hesitantly with frequent pausing
- staring. It is intimidating – the intimidated person evades eye contact or looks down, the nervous person looks away.

Dress codes

- What does your appearance say about the impression you wish to convey to others?
- Is your dress fussy or relaxed?
- Do you power dress? Do you need to?

Look at other managers you meet. What is it about them that suggests authority? There is an unspoken NHS dress code: take time to look critically at what each look conveys. Authority or seniority is usually understated with modern, minimalist, clean, straight lines and simple blocks of colour in expensive, good quality materials. Jackets, shirts, trousers and haircuts tend to be simple and formal. Clothes are always impeccably clean and pressed.

Our appearance says a lot about our mood and how we feel about ourselves, and appearance can, and does, change often from day to day, depending on our mood. Aim for a personal style to express your own individuality. Dress codes are relaxing in the workplace, but this may not obviate your need to boost your self-esteem by dressing in a particular way. Dress in a way that genuinely makes you feel comfortable and efficient.

Many women don't reflect the importance of their jobs in the way they look or act. Their style lags behind their titles. People won't see you as important unless you project that importance: they forget your accomplishments if you don't keep them informed.

- Recognise your achievements and take credit for them. It's a mistake to look upon your accomplishments as routine.
- Let other people's opinions of you do the talking, as in: 'I was asked to make the key speech at the practice managers' convention this year' or 'I'll be tied up next week because I'm heading the new PMS project'.
- Angle your stories to highlight the qualities with which you want to impress people. If you want to demonstrate your assertiveness you would say 'I negotiated my way through that situation and we both achieved outcomes we were happy with'.
- Self-publicise but don't brag – the latter boasts to boost their ego. Your goal is quite different: you are implementing a carefully calculated reporting system designed to let people know what you are doing so that they will give you the opportunity to do more.

Finally, remember that confidence and high self-esteem are indicated when you no longer need to conform to someone else's standard, so find your own style, which may be to be quieter and less assuming, but ruthlessly efficient.

References

1   LaRouche J and Ryan R (1984) *Strategies for Women at Work*. Counterpoint/Unwin Paperbacks, London.

2   Quillam S (2001) 12 Ways to stop taking the blame. *Good Housekeeping*. February, pp. 76–7. (www.thegoodbookguide.com/gh).

3   Bond A (1985) *Games for Social and Life Skills*. Hutchinson, London, pp. 67, 84, 93.

Further reading

Back K and Back K (1999) *Assertiveness at Work*. McGraw-Hill, London.

De Angelis B (1995) *Confidence: finding it and living it*. Hay House, New York.

Appendix A

Self-help exercises you can do to assist in your development

Exercise 1. Labels

Write down 12 things you believe about yourself.[3] Where have your labels come from?

- The early years of life? Relatives often repeat things to very young children about their looks, personality or behaviour.
- More recent experiences? Especially the comments of friends and people with power over us.

We may take on these labels because we feel too powerless to reject them. However, it is possible to reconsider these labels and to change them if you want to. Labels may make you feel:

- life is more simple and straightforward
- a sense of personal worth
- secure and comfortable
- you are given permission to avoid doing things because 'you are not like that'.

But labels can be dangerous:

- they can keep us in fixed patterns of behaviour ('I am unemotional and never express my anger') when it is justified and it might be better to reveal our feelings
- they can allow us to opt out of things we might otherwise do
- we can avoid new experiences ('I am not like that') because the proposed experience does not fit our labels.

When changing unwanted labels:

- choose a label which you do not like about yourself
- identify under what circumstances you behave as described by the label: Where, when and with whom? How often? Describe a typical situation
- decide what it is that you actually do or do not do which earns the label
- if you want to change any of the labels decide what you could do to make the label invalid.

Exercise 2. Improve self-awareness

Make a note of your five best points. They may be your attitudes, feelings or something you can do. At the same time think of situations where you have demonstrated these best points. Decide why you are shy about revealing them.

Exercise 3. Needs

Twenty needs which many people have are listed below.[3] What are your needs – to:

- have an exciting life?
- be told what to do?
- have times when things don't change?
- have a quiet life?
- be liked by others?
- help others?
- be part of a team?
- be a leader?
- do things on your own?
- look good?
- feel physically fit?
- like yourself?
- achieve things?
- give affection?
- be respected?

Which needs are most satisfied?
Which needs are least satisfied?
What can you do towards satisfying your least satisfied needs?

Exercise 4. Some ways to improve your understanding of non-verbal behaviour

In the following exercises, think about:

- eye contact
- seating positions
- loudness of voice
- tone of voice
- facial expression
- body posture.

Convey the following emotions to a partner. Can they guess the emotion? What leads them to think as they do?

- Openness
- Defensiveness
- Evaluating
- Suspiciousness
- Readiness
- Insecurity
- Cooperativeness.

Exercise 5

How do we behave when we are?

Excited	Puzzled	Frightened	Interested
Irritated	Depressed	Anxious	Surprised
Sarcastic	Critical	Bored	

Exercise 6

Think of three or four recent difficult encounters you have had with other people.

Situation	My verbal response	My body language	My feelings	What I really wanted to say/do	How I would have chosen to handle the situation assertively

CHAPTER 3

How to be assertive

Assertive communication is honest and direct; it is speaking your mind without fudging the issue or being aggressive. The assertive speaker is prepared to:

- be specific
- be honest and open
- negotiate
- repeat their message if misunderstood
- compromise if it is reasonable to do so
- listen
- self disclose: express their feelings
- innovate: take chances and risks
- accept criticism where appropriate
- prompt others to express themselves honestly.

Assertive communication usually leaves both speaker and listener feeling more comfortable than avoidance or confrontation.

Many working in healthcare are already skilled communicators as they are selected for their interpersonal communication skills. It is worth reflecting on some of your own skills.

Step one: understand yourself

- See if there is a pattern in the way you interact with people.
- Recognise assertiveness in yourself.
- Remember the times when something you did or said worked well.

To find out how you are likely to respond in a given situation, try the following exercises.

Exercise 1

Write a list of five situations in which you would like to behave more assertively. Then, next to each situation, note your current response – P = passive, A = aggressive or I = indirect (manipulative).

Exercise 2

For each of the following situations, ask yourself:

- What do you feel?
- Was your response aggressive, passive, assertive or manipulative?
- Which non-verbal behaviours were demonstrated?
- Describe and act out an assertive response.

1   A member of staff gives a blank 'no' when you make a request for them to attend training.
2   The senior partner interrupts your work by asking you to see a drug rep NOW, as he is unable to because his surgery is just beginning.
3   Your manager or one of the partners suddenly accuses you of attending too many meetings away from the practice/office – you are never available when needed. Is this a fair or unfair criticism?
4   A member of staff accuses you of talking behind their back about them. Is this a fair or unfair criticism?

Exercise 3

- List *who*, in friendships, work or family, makes you feel either passive or aggressive.
- List *when* you have behaved non-assertively (assertion being honest, direct, open communication).
- List *what* subjects make you feel and behave non-assertively, e.g. when making mistakes, discussing politics or expressing negative feelings.

Step two: learn about assertive behaviour

The following checklist gives a flavour of a style of communicating more honestly and directly. This leaves both parties feeling clearer and more comfortable with the interaction. The following ways of communicating are most helpful in difficult or problematic situations, e.g. when dealing with critical comments or manipulative behaviour, having to give criticism, or when negotiating.

Be clear and specific

- Think before you speak.
- Rehearse with sympathetic friends or colleagues.

- If the situation is problematic or awkward for you then you are more likely to hesitate or digress.
- Make the statement brief, and avoid unnecessary padding, especially when saying 'no' – 'sorry' and 'but' dilute the clarity and expose your uncertainty.
- Own your statement, assume responsibility.
- Keep your statement simple, brief and direct.

Example

'I have noticed that you have been late to work on several occasions over the last month, Pauline; tell me about why this is?'

Don't pass the buck; this diminishes your credibility and marks you as someone who is not willing to address the issue firmly.
   If you feel you are being criticised, but the criticism is messy, manipulative and nebulous, seek clarity yourself. No one likes giving criticism, so it is often done badly:

'I'm not sure if you really enjoy the organisational side of your job ... but the receptionists seem to like you.'

If this kind of comment is directed at you, ask for clarity:

'Last time we met you said you were unsure I liked the organisational side of my work. What makes you think that?' followed by: 'Let's look at ways we can change the situation'.

- Ask for clarification and examples to expose the criticism.

This allows both parties to identify the issue and begin to tackle it. Clarity untangles unexpressed needs, manipulation, sulking. When you express a willingness to both accept the situation and look at changing it, you regain the power.

Example

Sagarika has, on the whole, a good relationship with her manager, but occasionally she leaves an encounter feeling belittled and patronised. She is vaguely aware that she is being manipulated, and often feels criticised, but is finding it difficult to pinpoint. At her next meeting, she listens carefully to what her manager says to her, and finds that she is being subtly put down. Sagarika identifies feeling patronised, and, having identified this, is able to discuss her feelings with her manager.

Do not confuse clarity and directness with bluntness or rudeness. Being clear about an issue is being simple and intelligible about it. Clarity untangles unexpressed needs, manipulation, sarcasm or sulking. Being direct avoids the urge to whinge or complain, to respond in a roundabout way or reproach.

If you arrive in your office and find someone has used it in your absence and left it horribly untidy then tell them what you are unhappy about! Unless you tell them they will not know; they will not necessarily be able to see through your indirect sulks, nor may they correctly interpret them. Pinpoint the behaviour when it occurs.

Ask for clarification or 'read' behind the statement. Be *clear* in your own mind first what the issue is that you want to tackle.

Be open and honest about your feelings

- Tell how you feel, own it.
- Do not hide behind words.
- Do not use words to manipulate or hurt.
- Never say 'You make me feel' – no one can make us feel anything, we must take personal responsibility for our own feelings.
- Begin difficult situations with simple statements, for example 'I feel nervous/guilty/angry...'.

As we are rarely given the opportunity to explore negative feelings, this skill takes practice. To begin with, you may wish to notice the impact of your feelings physically, in your body, e.g. a sinking feeling, a lump in the throat, a tight chest or sickness. Name these, and then eventually you will feel more able to respond honestly and quickly.

Repeat your message

This technique is sometimes called the 'stuck record' or 'broken record' technique. If you feel misunderstood, or need to diffuse anger, calmly repeat your statement or request. By such gentle persistence you can maintain your position without falling prey to manipulative comment, irrelevant logic or argumentative bait. This is an especially useful skill to use when dealing with aggressive people:

- listen carefully to the other person's point of view
- acknowledge it
- then stick to your desired point
- repeat several times if necessary.

This will help you ignore the verbal traps that people sometimes set to draw us in. For example, 'I understand that you are feeling angry about the lack of appointments Mr Jones, this is something we are looking at and hoping to redress in the near future. I have logged your complaint'.

After hearing this three or four times the complainant gets the message. On the telephone, and as a last resort, try saying cheerfully and politely 'Thank you for calling!' before putting the phone down. This firmly closes the conversation.

This technique is best used in situations when your time and energy is precious, or when your rights are in danger of being abused. It is particularly useful when seeking a refund for faulty goods, or when you are refusing someone something and they persist. Be clear you are not going to give way.

Example A

In the following example Rebekah has just begun working on finalising the accounts when Dr X asks her to break off and see a drug representative.

Dr X: 'Oh, good, here you are. Here is Abdul from Bayer's. He has some information on a new product I'm interested in, and I'm in the middle of surgery. Can you have a word?'

Rebekah: 'I'm sorry I can't help right now, I've just started working on the accounts. Come in so we can make another appointment.'

Dr X: 'But this product is important – it represents big savings to the practice, can't you spare a little time?' (Manipulative bait – a plea to Rebekah's guilt.)

Rebekah: 'No, I wish I had the time.' (Repeats) 'I have a deadline to meet. Let's make it next Tuesday or Wednesday? I'd really like to hear about the product.'

Dr X: (critically) 'It won't take long, you know.' (Irrelevant logic.)

Rebekah: 'I understand it's frustrating for both of you (fielding the response and accepting some responsibility for the manipulative criticism) but I really need to finish this now.'

Dr X finally accepts Rebekah's refusal, and respects her determination and ability to set her own priorities. Rebekah has not been led by Dr X's own inability to manage his time, or aim to control her agenda. This classic situation is one where you are likely to be diverted by clever and articulate argument. Stay with what you need, relax and keep to your word. You may wish to alter the wording slightly each time, as Rebekah did, to avoid sounding artificial.

Example B

Liane, a registrar who has just completed a dermatology placement, is in her office and has just immersed herself in dictating her referrals when Dr M, the senior partner, knocks on the door in a fluster.

Dr M: 'Oh, Good, you've not yet left for visits. Can you come and see Mr Jones? I've just seen him and I want your opinion.'

Liane: 'I'm sorry I can't help, I've just started doing some paper work. I'll be able to see him next week when I've got a space. Let me look in my diary.'

Dr M: 'Oh. The problem is I can't start on treatment until I clarify this diagnosis. And he is pretty bad.' (Manipulative bait – a plea to the registrar's guilt.)

Liane: 'I understand that it's frustrating for both of you (fielding the response). I'll be able to see him next week.'

Dr M: 'It won't take long you know.' (Irrelevant logic.)

Liane: 'Yes, I know, but I need to do my paper work now. I've got a space next Tuesday at 10 o'clock. I'm able to see him then.'

Dr M finally accepts Liane's refusal.

This is a classic situation when you are likely to be diverted by clever, articulate, but irrelevant argument; or when you could lose your self-confidence if affected by the manipulative 'dig' to your self-esteem, provoking guilt.

One of the most effective things about using repetition in this way is that once you have prepared what you are going to say, you can relax and stay with your prepared argument. However manipulative or bullying the other person is, you know exactly what needs to be said.

There may be a situation when both parties are being assertive, in which case neither will want to continue for long, but work towards a compromise fairly quickly.

Fielding the response

This I consider as one of the most fundamental of all assertive skills. In order to successfully 'field' or 'fog' a response, you need to be able to indicate that you have heard what the other person has said without getting 'hooked' by what they say. Thus you are able to show that you respect the other person's point of view without necessarily sharing it. In order to communicate effectively, you need to listen, indicate that you have heard, acknowledge it, but stick to your guns. This skill is especially useful when handling direct or indirect criticism. The criticism may be direct, e.g.:

'You are never available when I want to see you', or implied
'Why can't Mr X have a home visit?'

In the second instance the request hides anger, frustration and resentment. You could 'read' behind the statement, so that your response could begin:

'I understand/accept that it must be very frustrating for you but ... I am unable to arrange a home visit ...' (offer an alternative).

Note that you need not be drawn into an explanation unless you choose to do so.

In the first instance, when the criticism is more direct, agreeing with the statement disarms your critic. You are acknowledging the probability that there may be some truth in what is said, while remaining your own judge – a powerful position. For example:

'Yes, I am often unavailable for you at short notice, however, I am still not able to deal with your request right now.'

Again, you do not need to justify your position.

Fogging, or fielding the response in this way allows you to receive criticism comfortably without becoming anxious or defensive. It also gives no reward to those manipulating you through unjustified criticism – people use criticism to diminish your self-esteem rather than in addressing the issue to help you understand yourself better.

When fielding you need to be emotionally intelligent and be aware of all the verbal and non-verbal messages that are being communicated or are leaking out. The other person needs to know that you understand their motives and feelings as well as thought. Listen out for the underlying issues, e.g.:

'You seem very angry/frustrated with me'
'I understand this is a difficult/upsetting situation'
'I accept that it must be very frustrating'.

Having shown that you are listening sympathetically, you are then able to continue confidently with your statement or answer; you are demonstrating that you are trying to understand the other person's point of view, but still hold your own:

'How come you can only see my child once a week for treatment when he needs it at least twice weekly?'

You read behind the statement and hear the anger and frustration of a concerned parent. Your response could begin:

'I accept that it must be very frustrating for you but ... I only hold this particular surgery once weekly.'

Note that you need not be drawn into an explanation unless you choose to.

Negotiate

- Be prepared to negotiate for what you want.
- Assertion does not mean always getting your own way!
- Cooperate, bargain as equals, work as a partnership towards achieving something you both want.

- Use tact and forethought.
- Empathise, cooperate, trade.
- Avoid confrontation.
- Seek the common ground.
- Aim for a win–win situation.

'I can see that you are unhappy about that, but I cannot complete the work today. I could finish it by Tuesday, though.'

'I understand that you need someone in post full time, but I did plan to only work for six sessions. Perhaps it would help if I spread those sessions over the whole week rather than working for three days on the trot?'

- Listen to the other party's point of view before you are able to bargain.
- Make certain that you fully understand the other person's position – ask for clarification if necessary.
- Prepare yourself well beforehand, harness the facts and figures that help you in supporting your case.
- Make certain that you keep to the point. If you feel the conversation is side tracking, bring the discussion back to the central issue: if necessary use the 'broken record' technique.

Effective negotiation should end with both parties coming to terms with a situation they both feel happy about and where neither one is compromised, but this does not always happen. Sometimes one party has to bow down. This does not necessarily mean that one of you has 'lost' if you do not get what you want. Reward yourself for making a courageous effort, and better luck next time!

Compromise

Compromise results when both parties have negotiated from an equal position. When moving towards a workable compromise a solution is found that takes the needs of both parties into consideration:

- give way to stubbornness
- do not wait for the other person to 'give in' first: offer a compromise
- bargain for material goods, but never compromise on your self-respect
- if you feel your personal worth is being questioned, respond as if you are being criticised
- remain objective and impartial.

There is no compromise about feelings: you have to respect another person's feelings as he or she does your own. Assertive behaviour is fair; there is no win/lose but a mutually successful outcome. To compromise is to concede, to meet half way. See if you can view compromise as making a virtue of necessity.

Accepting criticism

This skill helps you handle constructive criticism from others by agreeing with or accepting criticism if appropriate instead of reacting to it as if it were an accusation. Like self-disclosure, this allows you to look more comfortably at the less positive aspects or your own personality or behaviour without denying that that behaviour exists or becoming defensive. At the same time it reduces your critic's hostility. Examples of your response may be 'yes, I know I can be aggressive at times' and 'you are right, I am untidy'.

Only agree with the criticism if it is fair or truthful. If you acknowledge the probability of truth in their comment, it disarms the critic, and you demonstrate that you remain your own judge. If someone criticises you directly, learn to acknowledge and agree with the criticism, but only if you feel that the criticism is fair or truthful.

Expressing feelings

The importance of understanding and sharing feelings cannot be underestimated in any discussion on assertion.

- Learn to identify, or clarify, how we feel before responding to any situation.
- Learn to identify what your emotions are telling you.
- Talk about your feelings with another person.
- Share some of your vulnerability.

Personal exposure does carry a risk, but it is an important part of the openness and honesty of being assertive.

Prompting others to express themselves

This skill allows you to more comfortably seek out criticism about yourself, while prompting the other person to express negative feelings with more honesty. It can improve communication, especially in close relationships, and also encourages your critics to be more assertive. For example, if you suspect that the person you are talking to is hiding their true (negative) feelings, you may ask:

'Are you finding me difficult to talk to?'
'Do you think I am being unfair?'
'Does it seem as though I am pushing you into a corner again?'
'I hear you saying that you think I am disorganised, is that right?'

When behaving assertively, you are confronting issues and situations rather than waiting passively in the hope that you will be able to respond. It is less stressful, and more powerful, to set the agenda yourself.

There are times in any conversation when we suspect that there is something 'going on' beneath the surface. Often it is an intuitive feeling, or a suspicion that something is being said 'between the lines'. At times like this, follow your intuition and take the initiative to seek out, or prompt, an honest response.

Listen

- The assertive person listens carefully.
- Watch and listen to the actual statement, and also for an underlying message.
- Learn to 'read' behind the words, and also to watch non-verbal behaviour for 'leakage' or signs that all is not as it seems.
- Clarify or check that you have heard correctly – this is a good way of stalling for time before responding if you cannot identify how you feel about a situation:
  - 'So you think that I ought to be clearer about the facts?'
  - 'Can I just check what you just said ...?'

Active listening is a physically demanding, conscious process of attending to what the speaker is saying. It requires the receiver to listen for the total meaning a person conveys; to try to determine both the content of the message and the feelings underlining it. Active listeners note all the cues, both verbal and non-verbal, in communication.

Good listeners:

- *listen*: pay close, interested, attention
- *paraphrase*: demonstrate they have correctly perceived the sender's inner state and understood, e.g. 'Are you saying you dislike that kind of work ...?'
- *ask questions* to clarify the position, or reflect back that you have heard, e.g. 'So that made you feel very angry?'
- *never interrupt*
- *never advise* or suggest solutions
- *allow feelings*: they do not try not to stop them but encourage them – suppressing feelings will only increase the sender's discomfort and discourage them from trusting you.

See Appendix A for some exercises to improve your listening.

Innovate

- Take charge and regain control.
- Act as your own catalyst for change.
- Innovate and don't wait for others, or fate, to take over.

Some people find that once they are able to let themselves set the scene for change in this way, other areas of their life are affected; they have the confidence to move ahead and perhaps alter the balance of control in their personal as well as professional life. Once you allow yourself to be assertive, you are acknowledging that you are no longer the passive victim of other people's manipulation. You are able to make your own decisions, and this can be a very powerful motivator for change.

Empower

Assertiveness is a very powerful and freeing tool. When we behave assertively we experience very positive feelings, and those feelings inevitably become more meaningful, or central to our lives. Assertive behaviour gives us a certain strength and stability; it allows us to have more influence and authority. This extra power is very energetic and potent, but must be used wisely. It is very tempting after years of feeling oppressed or restricted to rush out and regain the world! Allow room for negotiation or compromise.

When we behave assertively it allows us to have more influence and authority within our professional role, and as human beings. In learning to be assertive you are releasing untapped potential and beginning a process of self-discovery through which you can begin to understand yourself, and others, more. Through being assertive you also empower others, allowing them the room to take space and negotiate their needs. As your sensitivity to others increases, so will your ability to feel care and compassion.

Use these skills wisely and recognise that the learning process is slow. Assertiveness is something that takes many, many years to effect; after all, you are learning to undo several years' worth of habitually different behaviour. So go slowly, and accept that in learning to be assertive you are beginning a process of self-discovery through which you can begin to understand your true potential. Some key points are to:

- be proactive
- begin with the end in mind
- take first things first – prioritise
- think win–win
- seek first to understand, then be understood.

If in doubt think:

- I think
- I feel
- I need
- I want.

Appendix A

Improve your listening skills

Participants work in pairs.

Exercise 1

- 'A' tells a partner of a true incident that happened to her.
- 'B' repeats it, trying to keep the same emphasis and reflection that 'A' had in the telling.
- 'A' takes on a different role (e.g. an absent-minded older woman) and tells the story again.
- Discuss the different impacts within each telling before swapping roles.

Exercise 2

One person explains for five minutes what they have been doing that day, or talks about their last holiday. The listener demonstrates (by giving verbal and non-verbal cues) that they are listening. They then change their behaviour to show that they are not listening.

- At the end of five minutes the partners swap roles and discuss how it felt to be in each position.
- Look at what kinds of behaviour indicate listening/not listening.
- What is assertive or aggressive about behaviour in this context?
- Discuss how people feel as recipients of each type of behaviour.

Exercise 3

Divide into pairs. Spend three minutes each on sharing information either about yourself or a cause you believe in and why.

- Summarise what was said.
- Listen to each other's summaries.
- Discuss any difficulties you had listening to each other, what outside interferences or mannerisms hindered your ability to listen.
- Give each other feedback on how they communicated verbally and non-verbally.
- Make the feedback constructive and specific, e.g. 'It would be better if you talked a little louder' rather than 'you talk too softly' or 'your voice wasn't right'.

CHAPTER 4

Feelings

In the last chapter we looked at the importance of identifying feelings clearly before responding to a situation. We need to look at why this skill is so important and why it is something that many of us find so difficult.

Notice how emotions tie up with a physical feeling. Think of when you feel you are understood, or have a choice. How do you feel when you are not loved or understood? Try and identify the physical feeling that goes with the emotion.

Exercise 1. How do you feel?				
FEELING	EMOTIONS	PHYSICAL	WITHOUT	FEELING
Loved	Happy/ confident	Warm/ energetic	Insecure/ rejected	Sick and tense
Understood				
Given choice				

Exercise 2

List all the positive and negative things you can think of about each of these people in turn:

Mother

Positive	Negative	I feel
Good sense of humour	Can be insensitive to my feelings	

Father

Positive	Negative	I feel
Generous	Very stubborn	

Sibling/friend

Positive	Negative	I feel

Dr/Mr/Ms Difficult at work

Positive	Negative	I feel
Thoughtful about patients	Thoughtless around staff	

Dr/Mr/Ms Easy

Positive	Negative	I feel

Are there any links? Similarities between people? What pushes your buttons the most?

To behave assertively we need to verbalise, act on, and hence release feelings. This is difficult for all of us in western cultures because:

- expression of feeling in adulthood is discouraged
- intellectual and rational behaviour predominate
- emotion or intuition are seen as 'female' and hence devalued in favour of the more rational 'male' states
- adults are supposed to be in control, so negative feelings are often suppressed to the detriment of our emotional and physical health.

Anne Dickson notes that feelings are physiological events that happen inside our bodies, but 'we talk of becoming "overpowered" by rage or "beside ourselves" with anger, which reinforces the idea that these feelings are somehow detached from us'.[1] Feelings actually generate changes in our body chemistry. Symptoms such as a lump in the throat, a pounding heart, sinking stomach or sweaty palms mean that our body is communicating effectively and we can build on that.

Some facts about feelings

- **We can't be held responsible for our feelings, as we can't stop our body reacting, but we can take charge of how we act on those feelings.**

We can verbalise and share feelings; telling others when we feel sad, angry, envious or unsure. Although people can argue with your logic, they cannot deny or dismiss your feelings. You have a right to them.

It is thought that feelings that are not released can accumulate, leading to stress-related illness. Any work on releasing feelings (for example, in psychotherapy) is very cathartic and freeing. There is some debate about the usefulness of releasing feelings physically, but there is no harm in naming the feeling appropriately. If you are provoked to anger during a meeting, it may be appropriate to simply say you are feeling angry until you are able to release the anger physically – by punching a cushion, perhaps, in a safer environment. Feelings can be diffused: if you understand and acknowledge them, it helps to release and dissipate the chemical build up.

- **By verbalising feelings, one takes a risk and shares something very personal, and there is a high chance that others will be freed up to do the same. This personal exposure enhances and builds relationships.**
- **Feelings often conflict with what we think is rational.**

If your present reaction seems inappropriate, you could be responding to something unresolved from your past. It may help to understand what is behind the feeling: sadness or loss? If, for example, your parents were over-critical when you were young, it may be especially difficult for you to accept criticism from authority figures now. Here you need to identify and not dismiss the feeling in the hope it will go away. Correct identification of a feeling such as humiliation or anger can lead to its resolution.

- **We need to be able to make choices in our lives.**

If this need is blocked we experience frustration, helplessness, irritation and anger. If the need is fulfilled, we feel powerful, enthused and energised. One of the reasons why morale is so low in the clinical professions at present is because that need to make choices and change things is being cramped by government dictates. There is frustration with a lack of funding, time and unsympathetic or badly informed management. We are all familiar with the feelings of helplessness and outrage that result.

- **We need to feel understood.**

If this need is satisfied we feel secure, safe and valued. If not, feelings range from feeling isolated and fearful to anxious, panicky and confused. If we feel our role is misunderstood at work, we seek support and understanding from colleagues in the same profession. The depth and quality of that feeling varies depending on how much we identify with our work.

- **We have a need to give and receive love and friendship.**

Once this need is fulfilled we experience closeness, belonging and affection. If it is denied us, the negative feelings are sadness, rejection and loneliness. Many of us get a great deal of satisfaction from working as a member of a close-knit team. If the team is not cohesive, or you work much of the day in isolation, disharmony of feeling can result.

Three levels of expression

Psychologists discuss how feelings can be expressed at three different levels:[2,3]

- acknowledgement
- verbal expression
- physical release.

At the *first level*, you may choose to privately notice and acknowledge what you feel, without verbalising it. Many people experience a time lapse between the experience of an emotional response and the acknowledgement of it. Often the realisation comes later, with a flash of recognition; 'If only I'd said such and such!' With time you will become more adapt at recognising what is going on, and learn to act on it quickly.

At the *second level* you may make a simple statement about how you feel: 'I feel very happy/envious', 'That makes me feel very angry', 'I feel hurt by that comment'. The immediate effect of this is to reduce your anxiety, allowing you to relax and take control.

At the *third level* feelings are released physically. You need to find your own way of releasing anger: yelling in the car on the way home; punching a cushion, any way that you find easy to release that frustration. Crying can be a very therapeutic way to release pent-up disappointment or sadness; allow yourself to mourn. Use the information your body is giving you to release the emotions in a safe place.

Feelings are powerful, and negative feelings especially provoke fear. Because we fear their intensity, we often try to harness them, to control them, in order to somehow diminish their power. But once you allow yourself to feel them, they lose their power. Ride with it. Once you have experienced the feeling fully it no longer controls you, it becomes something familiar and therefore less scary. If you cut yourself off from what you feel not only is this psychologically dangerous, but you are denying yourself access to your wise inner self and closing the door to self-expression and fulfillment.

Dealing with the emotions

Anger

- Anger can be positive, powerful and energising.
- There is a general taboo in western society on the expression of anger.
- We equate anger with aggression, arrogance and unfemininity.
- Anger can motivate us to change things, it gives us the impetus to move direction in life or take up challenges.
- Anger can be vigorous, creative and determined.
- Anger makes politicians, charity leaders and many of society's leading figures.
- Anger makes doctors, nurses and therapists.

Where we feel angry, we care, and we are motivated to change things. Where anger is devalued it gets suppressed, and it remains for many people one of the most difficult emotions to handle. For middle and 'owning' (upper) class men and women, it is especially difficult to reveal that side of their nature. These social groups are, from childhood, encouraged to repress 'difficult' (especially noisy) emotions: to be 'ladylike', compassionate and caring. Often it is the woman's experience to be told that such behaviour is threatening or domineering; men often equate our anger with hysteria. Because we have not been allowed to experience anger, we fear its effects, and imagine that being angry is like unleashing a wild dog that will provoke violence, and destroy everything in its path.

What happens when we block our anger?

- It emerges as aggression which is a form of badly stifled anger.
- We repress it still further and respond passively or not at all.
- A non-response blocks the energy, and the power moves within, holding us back.
- This form of control leads us to build up hurtful feelings.
- Helplessness leads quickly to apathy, resignation and depression.

It is possible to understand and express your anger assertively. Acting to revoke those feelings of resentment and powerlessness can create change in your own life. Once we allow ourselves to express anger we recall some of that energy and regain a sense of our own power and purpose.

The different faces of anger

We employ a variety of ways through which we express anger indirectly:

- we flare under the slightest provocation, showing that hurt and frustration has been slowly accumulating beneath the surface
- we control ourselves and anger eventually emerges as sarcasm or bullying
- we bury it, whine or moan
- we feel irritable, frustrated, tense, spiteful or resentful
- we feel impotent, constrained or aggrieved.

How to communicate feelings assertively

1 *Identify the feeling.* Begin by identifying the feeling. Watch for the signs that your body gives: Do you feel a rush of adrenalin? Do you feel hot, sweaty, sick, frightened or powerful?

2 *Are you on safe ground?* Check that you feel safe enough to express your feeling. If not, take steps towards controlling them temporarily. Allow yourself the time and space afterwards to release the frustration.

3 *Confront the source of the feelings.* Try and identify whether you are managing immediate and direct feelings in a situation, or whether you are reacting to past hurts and stresses. If the latter applies you still need to look at:
    - what is causing the feelings to surge up
    - how you can alleviate the problem.

4 *Verbal statement.* Try a simple statement: 'I am angry', 'That makes me feel very angry'. This immediately diffuses much of the tension.

5 *Watch the non-verbals.* Anger often makes women cry, which can infuriate men. It may be that women have learned to cry for sympathy, so hoping

to diffuse the situation or confuse, and hoping people will forget the anger and concentrate instead on the sadness. Or more likely, it is perhaps the only way they were allowed as a child to express deep felt emotion. Boys and men, on the other hand, are allowed to be angry and show aggression more freely, but are not allowed to cry.

- Watch that you don't smile nervously, use sarcasm or sneer.
- Check that your tone of voice and body movements match what you are saying. Remember that a small, tight or little-girl voice does not carry with it the same conviction as a deeper, louder adult one.

Exercise 3.

- List five things that make you feel *angry*, e.g. 'people who swear'.
- List five things that make you feel *hurt*, e.g. 'people who ignore me'.
- List five things that make you feel *happy*, e.g. 'people who respect my need for privacy'.
- List five things that make you feel *irritated*, e.g. 'people who push in a queue'.

References

1   Dickson A (1982) *A Woman in Your Own Right*. Quartet Books, London.

2   Ellis A (1979) (Audio cassette) *RETR and Assertiveness Training*. Albert Ellis Institute for Rational-Emotive Behaviour Therapy, New York.

3   Beck AT, Rush AJ, Shaw BF and Emery G (1979) *Cognitive Therapy of Depression*. Guilford, New York.

CHAPTER 5

Making and refusing requests

Saying no

Exercise 1

List those things that you do for other people because they ask you, not because you want to do them. List under work, friendship and home:

Work	Friendship	Home

Swap lists with a friend and then try role-playing. Practice saying 'no' politely, e.g. 'Can I borrow your car please?', 'No, Antonio, I never lend my car to anyone but family. Why don't you try hiring one?'

Exercise 2

Consider the following:
- Do you instantly respond with a 'yes' if you are asked a favour at home or work?
- Are you setting yourself up to be a super-manager/doctor/therapist/nurse?
- Or do you feel comfortable refusing requests, and can you live with the guilt that may follow?

We have already discussed how women especially find it easy to get caught up in this scenario. Culturally, women are taught to be selfless and caring. They are taught to readily give up their own needs in order that someone else feels comfortable. They are taught, both overtly and subtly, that their own needs should come last. This behaviour can, of course, have a pay off in terms of power; by being seen to 'do it all' and cope marvellously, women are in fact clawing back some of the power that is unevenly distributed between the sexes.

General practices all over Britain resound with the cry: 'No, no, don't help; it's quicker if I do it!'. The offer of help is tactfully withdrawn and the super-person regains the 'power' over her domain. She has the knowledge, the authority and the ability. In her surgery she rules. This struggle with delegation occurs at home with the children too – women feel it is easier, and better, to do it themselves. Maybe it is, in the short term, but others suffer from not feeling empowered and learning from the experience; and the super-person burns out with overwork.

It takes great effort to relinquish some of that power. Making that choice can be very freeing, but it can also cause some internal conflict, as the adult woman is taking a stand against the child within her, and that new role takes time to nurture and grow.

In delegating, the manager reaps new rewards and gains a different power that is non-manipulative. She learns more about the power of equality and of real choice. She learns to be assertive, and she learns to share.

Women are socialised to be compliant and to win approval. It can be very difficult to throw off that innate dependence and continuing need for (parental) approval; but it is not impossible. When we become an adult we can, and do, make our own choices in life; by saying 'no' for ourselves we are rejecting the underlying need to be liked; we choose for ourselves.

Consider some of the work situations in which it is difficult to make a refusal.

- A PCT manager is pressing you for some information that is confidential to your practice.
- You are seeing a patient to talk through a complaint. The conversation drifts away from the subject in hand towards another problem they have. You feel sorry for the patient and flattered that you are being asked for advice. It becomes increasingly hard to end the conversation.
- You are approached and asked if you could give a lift home to the senior partner's two children, who live near to you, but in fact not in the direction you usually take. You are pressed for time as you have an evening commitment.
- You are invited to a colleague's retirement party on an evening that clashes with your child's open evening at school.

Having acknowledged that it is difficult, but not impossible, for women to move out of the compassion trap, let us look at some of the common misconceptions about saying 'no'.

'Saying "no" directly is rude and blunt'

Because we are unused to saying 'no' without padding or excuses, we tend to feel that it is impolite, but a 'no' can be said politely, and with respect:

- take responsibility for your decision
- allow the other person space to express their feelings
- practise saying 'no' clearly and directly, without padding, frills or apology
- do not elaborate, offer excuses or explanation; you do not need to
- take responsibility for saying no, rather than blaming someone else
- acknowledge their problem, but stay with your answer – no:
  - 'I can see your predicament, but I can't help you'
  - 'I know that it will be difficult for you to find someone else for the evening, but no, I can't help you out tonight'.

'Saying "no" is selfish, uncaring and mean'

By saying 'no' you are being clear about your own wishes and needs, and people will respect you for this honesty. When someone asks you to do something you do not have to respond. Remind yourself when you last asked someone for a favour, or to spend time with you on a project, or to provide cover for you, and they refused. No doubt you accepted their refusal without question. Allow yourself the same freedom and respect that you give others:

- your own needs are important
- your own needs are no more or less important than anyone else's, but of equal import
- saying no more frequently will allow you to begin to balance your own needs with that of other people.

This is not self-preoccupation or narcissism, but a description of balanced care, extended with the same concern to self as others. In saying 'no' you are setting new limits for yourself; you are giving yourself adequate time to rest and replenish your energy, to enable you to make more active choices on how you spend your time. People rarely admire or respect someone who thinks so little of herself that she never gives herself time. Remember that when we are intent on being selfless, we easily become over-stretched and exhausted by our responsibilities – at great cost to our physical and mental well-being.

'People won't like me if I say "no"'

Will people really think you selfish or greedy if you say no? In fact, the reverse is often true: people respect you for being clear about your own limitations. Also, because you are more in control of yourself and your own time, you respect yourself more as well. When you acknowledge any negative feelings that you feel the other person has about your refusal, there should be no reason for their dislike. An assertive 'no' should leave both parties feeling comfortable. If we suppress a lot of our negative feelings in order to gain love and respect, we deny that we have any needs. We then do all that is asked of us but end up saying 'no' indirectly, in a begrudging way.

'Saying "no" will cause others to take offence. It will make them feel rejected and hurt'

You are refusing the *request* not the *person* when you say 'no'. If you anticipate that your 'no' will be hurtful in some way, remember to acknowledge that.

'Disagreement and conflict are a disaster and must be avoided at all costs'

- Not so. Everyone we meet is unique and likely to hold different views.
- It can be very refreshing, intellectually and emotionally, to discuss these differences.
- Conflict can be painful, but we learn through its resolution.

Being assertive opens up new lines of communication. Your honesty allows the other person equal space to be honest, so the disagreement, if there is one, is brought out into the open and dealt with there.

Other ways of saying 'no'

- Learn to notice your immediate 'gut response' when a request is made. Try and identify reactions which signal uncertainty, doubt or uneasiness. If you experience these, your answer should be 'no'.
- If in doubt, allow yourself to hesitate. You are not obliged to make an instant decision; give yourself breathing space before committing yourself. Acknowledge your uncertainty and ask for qualifying information about what the commitment would entail if you agreed to the request:
  - 'If I were to accept, what would my responsibilities be?'
  - 'I think I would like to do it, but I need time to think. I'll get back to you by next Wednesday.'
  - 'If I said yes, would you be able to support me if x, y, or z happened?'
- If the person making the request tries to draw you into debate or asks you to change your mind, repeat your refusal calmly and clearly. Try using the 'stuck record' technique. Use the same wording exactly and they will soon respect your resolve.

- Take responsibility for saying no, do not blame someone else, and do not apologise.
- Check your body language:
  - make sure you look the person in the eye, as you say 'no'
  - try moving away or making a 'no' hand movement if the 'no' is final and blunt
  - check that you are not smiling apologetically as you talk and maintain firm eye contact
  - sit or stand upright and keep your voice steady and clear.
- Change the conversation afterwards to avoid lingering on what may be perceived as an unpleasant topic.
- Identify your immediate feelings and acknowledge the difficulty honestly:
  - 'It's difficult for me to say this, but no'
  - 'I feel uncomfortable saying this, but the answer is no'.
- Use 'I' language to show that you have a strong belief in your own judgement, convictions and decisions.
- Don't overuse fillers: 'I'm sorry', 'Please', 'Excuse me'. The overapologetic person will say, 'Excuse me, I'm so sorry I interrupted you'. Compare this with the considerate response, 'I can see you're busy. Would tomorrow be a good time?'.

Remember that you are refusing the request, not rejecting the person. Saying 'no' and surviving the guilt does get easier with practice!

Exercise 3

Stand opposite a friend. One of you says 'yes' to their opposite partner, the other side says 'no', loudly and firmly.

Exercise 4

Reply assertively to the questions from this list. Swap roles and discuss how it feels to be the recipient of a firm 'no'. Practice saying 'no' assertively, without apology or aggression.

- 'Would you like to stay for a cup of tea, my daughter's arriving and she'd love to meet you?'
- 'Can you pop this document into Rachel's house on your way home? I haven't got a car today?'
- 'Can you give Christopher an extra 20 minutes treatment today as I have a hospital appointment and I won't be back until 5.00 pm?'
- 'Can you be quick on that phone as I need to use it?'
- 'Do you mind if you see your patients in this room today as we are holding an exhibition in the room you usually use?'
- 'Can I borrow this book?'
- 'Can I borrow your car please – I have got visits to do and mine is right out of petrol?'
- 'Have you got a minute?'
- 'Can you take a stint on reception, Moira is away and they are very rushed?'
- 'Can you sort out the light bulb in the toilet, it's gone again?'
- 'Someone's been sick in the waiting room – the nurses are busy so can you clear it up?'
- 'You will need to change that meeting date as I've got to drive Lilly to her violin lesson.'
- 'There's no need to go to that meeting.'

Making requests

Learn to ask for what you want with clarity and without aggression. You have a right to make your wants known to others, and they have the right to say no!

Ask for what you want:

- specifically and directly. If you ask indirectly or drop hints, you run the risk of not being heard, or being misunderstood and your request may go unheeded as a consequence
- clearly and honestly. Practice asking for what you want without guise. Instead of: 'I suppose I ought to go and make the coffee' (begrudging); or: 'Why is it always me that makes the coffee?' (whining); try: 'Pramita, can you make the coffee today please?' Or, instead of looking for support amongst your colleagues about how your boss does not understand the concept of working women. 'Can we make the meeting a little earlier to

give those of us with children plenty of time to set off?' People will not know automatically or through telepathy how difficult you are finding it all unless you tell them.

Learn to take charge of a situation and give yourself the permission and authority to ask for what you want.

Checklist on making requests

- Be specific – do not drop hints.
- Be honest.
- Take charge of the situation.

CHAPTER 6

Dealing with conflict

Preventing and resolving conflict

In all work situations, there will be conflicts that should be avoided, and conflicts that should be managed. Possible approaches to *preventing* conflicts include:[1]

- recognising and accepting differences between individuals and groups, in terms of values, perceptions, expectations and needs
- being honest with oneself, and with others
- allocating sufficient time and energy to really get to know the people you work with, so that you understand their values, beliefs, etc.
- not automatically assuming that you are right and they are wrong
- not feeling defensive if others disagree with your ideas
- providing suitable ways in which people can express their feelings about things
- ensuring that people learn from previous conflicts that have been resolved.

Resolving conflicts at work

Where it is not possible to prevent a conflict occurring, then it may become necessary to try to resolve it in as positive and constructive a manner as possible. Successful conflict resolution has to be based on an accurate and thorough understanding of the actual conflict itself. There are five broad approaches that can be taken for successful conflict resolution. The approach adopted should match the particular characteristics and circumstances of the conflict situation.

- *Denial*. Trying to solve the conflict by withdrawing and denying its existence. This can be satisfactory if the conflict is relatively unimportant, or if there is a need for a cooling-off period before the conflict is tackled head-on.

- *Suppression.* Differences are played down and a harmonious façade is constructed. Again, this approach can be satisfactory for relatively unimportant conflicts, or for situations where the relationship between the two parties in conflict must be preserved at all costs.
- *Domination.* The conflict is resolved by one party using their authority or position. This approach can be satisfactory where the domination is based on clear authority or where the approach has been agreed upon by the parties involved.
- *Compromise.* Resolution occurs when each party gives something up in order to meet halfway. This approach can be satisfactory if both parties have sufficient room to alter their positions, although overall commitment to the 'agreed upon' solution may be in doubt.
- *Collaboration.* Individual differences are recognised and the aim is for group consensus, so all participants feel that they have won. This approach can be satisfactory if there is the time available and the individuals believe in the approach and have the necessary skills.

Handling conflict

Conflicts are part of normal everyday life; too few, and life is boring, too many and life can become stressful. Conflicts are nearly always caused by people having different points of view, or by people trying to achieve what they want at the expense of others. Some of the principal causes of conflict at work are:

- misunderstandings
- personality clashes
- differences in goals/methods to be used
- substandard performance
- problems relating to areas of responsibility and authority
- lack of cooperation
- frustration
- competition for limited resources
- non-compliance with rules and policies.

Many managers spend too much time at work dealing with conflict. However, there are positive and negative aspects of conflict in organisations.

Conflict can be positive when it:

- helps to open up discussion of an issue
- results in problems being solved
- increases the level of individual involvement and interest in an issue
- improves communication between people
- releases emotions that have been stored up
- helps people to develop their abilities.

Conflict can be negative when it:

- diverts people from dealing with the really important issues
- creates feelings of dissatisfaction among the people involved
- leads to individuals and groups becoming insular and uncooperative.

Conflicts that are likely to result in positive outcomes are to be encouraged in organisations, and negative-outcome conflicts have to be either prevented or resolved in a positive manner.

Over the years, most managers will have developed a number of approaches to such situations, based on their own experiences. The effective manager is one who is able to draw upon a wide range of approaches and is able to apply them to situations that are fully understood. Understanding the nature and causes of conflict at work, and being able to use a wide range of approaches to prevent and resolve conflict, are essential for anyone with managerial responsibilities.

Dealing with patient complaints

The best way of dealing with complaints or provocative or aggressive behaviour is to be proactive, so you both minimise the complaints and prepare ahead for their resolution. The maxim is to:

- keep patients informed
- provide the very best service you can afford
- respect patients' wishes for clean, tidy, private and well kept premises
- display any relevant policies and procedures, e.g. complaints, repeat prescriptions, and supply a system for informing patients about delays
- make certain that records are available when the patient consults
- audit complaints and plaudits, categorise the reason for the failure and be open about naming the person responsible, collectively discuss ways to solve the problem, and implement them
- give patients copies of correspondence relating to them along with a glossary of medical abbreviations and terms
- train all staff to be welcoming, attentive and helpful, and to keep negative opinions to themselves.

Common negative patient experiences are usually due to *poor communication*:

- with patients
- with other professionals
- within the system
- due to variations in provisions
- due to poor information
- because of a lack of understanding/acknowledgement of the real emotional issues affecting the patient and carers
- due to bureaucracy and hierarchies benefiting the system not patients.

Any good initiative has at its root good, or better, communication between patient, professionals and staff. Look at the following recent initiatives and note who benefits most, and why.

- NSFs.
- Local centres of excellence.
- Collaborative care planning.
- Patient forums.
- Primary/secondary care protocols.
- More screening/assistance for carers.
- Individual and local initiatives, e.g. taped consultations in cancer care.

Despite our best efforts, many of our patients do experience problems within the system, and complain. When this happens, the role of the manager within the practice is not to ignore, but pull together the evidence and present it back to his or her team so it can inform future, better practice.

According to a recent report from the GMC, the most common complaints needing resolution from general practice are associated with poor communication: inappropriate or ineffective care management, or the complainer having some association with grief, or delayed or failed diagnosis.[2]

Some solutions

- Say sorry if you're in the wrong.
- Speak directly to the complainant – an apology given over the telephone results in a higher level of complaints being resolved than apology by letter.
- Put the problem right immediately – do not cause the patient further delay or anguish.
- Your response must be real and important to you, otherwise it will be perceived as a standard and impersonal business response:
  - apologise first, explaining who is responsible without apportioning specific blame
  - acknowledge the patient's anxiety using clear language
  - acknowledge and understand the problem you have caused them
  - then give an explanation, but only if it is essential
  - finish with how you are going to put it right
  - thank the complainer for drawing your attention to the matter.

Example

A patient telephones the practice to change a date with the practice counsellor. The message is relayed wrongly and the patient subsequently arrives expecting to see the counsellor, who is absent on that day.

Dear Ms Blank

I do apologise on behalf of the practice for the mix-up regarding your cancellation, which meant that we did not get to meet today. It must have been very difficult to arrive and find I was not there. Unfortunately, I understood the cancellation referred to X date. I am so sorry that our work was unexpectedly disrupted. The practice will of course give you a further session. I look forward to seeing you again on Y.

How to handle difficult patients or situations

How do you react when you are worried and panicky? It may be that you can remain reasonable and considerate most of the time, but break under difficult circumstances. If the patient is *frightened* they need:

- privacy
- acknowledgement of their distress
- sympathetic handling
- firm reassurance
- your competence.

If they are *incompetent* they need you to:

- take charge
- clarify essential details, e.g. name, telephone number, address
- show compassion and kindly help
- not spell out the rules.

If the patient is *deeply distressed* and you have the unhappy task of communicating unwelcome news, try these ideas.[3] Bad news is to be shared not broken, as what is broken cannot be mended.

- Think about body language, eye contact, and language use.
- Never use euphemisms – they make communication unclear and misunderstandings will happen.
- Be clear, direct and honest.
- Look people in the eye.
- Sit next to or close to the person.
- If necessary, back up the news by reading any related correspondence together – people forget when distressed, and so remembering seeing it written down reinforces the point.
- Tape important conversations.
- Communicate honestly and without defence: patients and relatives have a right to know.

- Keep checking that you have been understood.
- Where possible make use of psychologists and counsellors to supervise and debrief, not doctors.
- Do not use humour and flippancy to defend yourself against the feelings – you are not the one that needs the defences.

Defensive behaviour

Avoid triggering defensive behaviour by:

- controlling
- blaming
- judging
- indifference
- giving misinformation.

Crying and loss of control

- Wait, do not offer verbal sympathy or intervene as this might escalate the situation.
- Say 'Let's take a moment to collect our thoughts'.
- Use sympathetic body language, e.g. three fingers on the side of the chin, head tilted to one side.

The chronic complainer[1]

- Ask for cooperation.
- Use positive language: 'If we don't cooperate there will be problem'.
- Is there anything I can say or do that would gain your cooperation?
- Plan ahead: 'So what do you want to see happen?'.
- Take control: 'I know what you have to say is important, but I can't listen at the moment. Can we take the issue to the next staff meeting and try and solve it there?' or 'I want to make sure I understand you – let's meet tomorrow when I have more time'.
- Try being silent, stop giving feedback.

Anger and aggression
The psychology of hate

Inappropriate and often violent expressions of anger and aggression are on the increase in our society, and we need to employ techniques to both effectively control our own anger and cope with other people's.

Some facts about anger are that:[5]

- anger affects our bodies, health and minds
- it is physically impossible to be relaxed and angry at the same time
- there is a connection between anger and depression
- we cannot think straight when we are angry
- venting the anger does not make it go away – it can make it worse
- uncontrolled anger is an emotionally driven trance state
- it is possible to learn to see things from a different perspective
- it is possible to inoculate yourself against stress build-up
- anger – and the build-up of the stress hormone cortisol – can have a devastating impact on your immune system and long-term health.

An uncontrolled/aggressive reaction is most common in all of us when we feel under threat, usually as a result of criticism. We react instantly; we rise to the bait easily and use defensive behaviour to deflect the comment in our defence. This sort of reaction is never constructive and can lead quickly to a heated argument. This is not an appropriate way to behave in a work situation, but it can and does occur. If you find things have developed in this way, there is a need for apology on both sides, one to acknowledge the provocation and one for reacting in such an uncontrollable way.

Anger is engendered by our expectation of unacceptable behaviour on the part of others. Our attitudes and behaviour are shaped by:

- experience
- beliefs
- needs
- values
- socioeconomic variances
- attitudes of others towards us.

Thus, there will always be a mismatch between what each of us considers acceptable behaviour. The aim is to try and understand each other's world, and find common ground.

What do we know and assume about anger? First, check out your prejudices, value systems and trust of others with this self-analysis questionnaire:

Exercise 1

1   What do people most frequently consult with in healthcare systems? Mental health problems? Problems related to long-term chronic disabilities? Why is it we are often reluctant to provide a service for these groups of people, given they make up the work we choose to do?

2   What would it take for you to leave your family, friends and culture and go and live in a place where you knew nobody, did not speak the language, and were not permitted to work? What qualities do you think you would need to do so? Stamina? Drive? Bravery? Do we equip asylum seekers with these qualities? Why not?

3   When you notice people in shopping malls, do you think:
    a)   some of them are just wandering around since they have nothing better to do?
    b)   they are shopping, exercising, or visiting with friends?

4   When a person with you speaks slowly, do you:
    a)   listen until the person finishes talking?
    b)   cut them off and finish off their statement?

5   When you are a front seat passenger, do you:
    a)   stay alert and watchful?
    b)   relax and enjoy the view?

6   When you notice someone in a restaurant who is obese, do you:
    a)   acknowledge she may have a physical or psychological problem?
    b)   wonder why she can't control her food intake?

7   While your partner is cooking dinner, do you:
    a)   keep them company and chat about your day while waiting?
    b)   occasionally check in on them to see what they are doing and make sure it doesn't overcook?

Reasons for anger

It is stressful when dealing with other's unwanted emotions. Oliver James has described how self-hatred can turn towards others.[4] Many health and care workers become 'dustbins' for their clients' anger and self-hatred. Clients/patients may unconsciously project these unwanted feelings in a covert or overt way: by missing appointments, keeping professionals waiting for appointments, or making veiled suicide threats.

Flows of aggression and depression run in families – we pass or dump from one to another, and get rid of our own angry, critical feelings by inducing them in another, thus moving from an 'I'm not OK, you are OK' position to 'I'm OK, you're not'.

It is thought that murderers stab or smash feelings held inside themselves into their victims. Rapists ejaculate their 'badness' into women, and those who commit or attempt suicide plague their loved ones with guilt, depression and rage: 'Look what you've made me do'. Both those who kill, and kill themselves, are thus paralysed by self-loathing.

James cites that three-quarters of convicted violent men are depressed, and become more depressed and aggressive when locked up. Depression can make those with aggressive tendencies violent to their partners and others. There is a fluidity of depression/aggression, where the pain is felt and then passed back.

How do we respond to anger?

We are frightened of anger, and our fear causes us to react in one of many defensive ways:

- *we ignore* – we speak in a bright and cheerful voice which forces the patient to push down and suppress the distress quickly
- *we placate* – we avoid eye contact, give a too-pleasant smile, and agree with the patient or give way to their demands
- *we are over-knowledgeable* – we try to blind the patient with science, using long words and explanations, insisting if the patient does as we say everything will be alright
- *we control* – keeping the patient at bay with distance and rank, quoting rules and regulations, insisting on specific behaviour or controlling the time allocation strictly
- *we respond angrily* – we react to their distress with loudness and strong gestures, bring in staff reinforcements, and accuse the patient of being a trouble-maker.

Does any of this help? If you, or a staff member, is faced with a difficult patient, the following trouble-shooting tips may help:

- make sure that the most appropriate member of staff is dealing with the situation: the one who feels least threatened, not necessarily the most senior
- match the patient's emotion rather than contradicting it – if they are angry, use a strong voice, if scared, drop your voice
- if extreme violence threatens, never leave it too late to call for help – make sure one member of staff on each shift has the responsibility for calling the police the minute trouble starts, otherwise everyone will think this is someone else's job

- if in doubt, leave the room taking other patients and staff with you. Equipment can be replaced – people can't.

People who behave reactively are out of control, they are responding to external influences. These reactive responses are related to *insecurity, unmet needs* and *fear*, so these feelings can be negated by asking:

'How secure do you feel here?'
'Are you getting what you need from us?'
'What are you scared of?'

Instead you should aim to:

- choose a response
- respond, not react
- look for a win–win outcome.

If we have a good self-image and self-esteem, we are able to think kindly of ourselves: 'I am someone who is thoughtful, caring and who has integrity'. Not everyone is able to do this. Good self-esteem helps us to behave assertively in difficult situations; we respect the needs of others and ourselves; we care enough to have the courage to connect. If we have awareness of, and commitment to, what we are doing, we understand enough of ourselves and are 'big' enough to behave with humility. If focused on our own ego we would behave:

- arrogantly
- greedily
- competitively
- in a self-focused way.

Perceptions that precipitate anger

- No-one likes me.
- I must be perfect.
- Everyone must follow my rules.

Conflict will always occur when there is miscommunication, conflict between personality types, differing values, perceptions and opposing objectives. Stress occurs when our perception colours an event that has triggered us emotionally. We are more likely to react angrily if stressed. In both instances, we need to find the common ground.

Strategies to reduce anger

When a patient confronts angrily:

1   acknowledge the situation
2   state your feelings
3   talk priorities
4   offer alternatives
5   use the broken record technique.

Do not:

* strut about
* point
* raise your voice.

Braithwaite has some additional ideas:[5]

* when shocked, we breathe rapidly: so relax, breathe deeply to signal non-aggression
* use open, free-flowing hand movements, one at a time
* read and avoid hand to head signals. These show signs of anxiety, loss of patience or can have sexual connotations
* do not fold your arms to form a barrier
* stand or sit at a slight angle, make use of good personal space
* do not touch: poking and pushing will escalate into serious assault, repetitive head nods are negative
* keep your face in tune: if you smile inappropriately it will be read as a smirk
* establish eye contact but be aware that some cultures do not establish eye contact with people they regard as superior
* reflective body language works in counselling, but not in aggressive situations
* be aware of gender, culture and ethnicity differences. Discuss differences openly to learn more; interpret correctly and react appropriately.

To avoid conflict escalation:

* listen
* remain calm and centred, detached from the personality
* focus on the facts rather than the position
* create and maintain a positive atmosphere
* consider 'time out'
* identify the needs and benefits of resolution
* agree where disagreements can coexist
* look for common ground
* aim for win–win.

Sometimes, no matter how effective the strategies are, the other person may choose not to resolve the conflict. If so, ask yourself:

- Is this conflict serious enough to end the relationship?
- Can I live with this constant conflict?
- What about when it's your supervisor, colleague, superior?

If the patient leaves the room angrily:

- do a self-analysis of the consultation: is there anything you could have done differently?
- act quickly to get back in control
- be positive
- retrieve the patient yourself
- invite them to sit down – it is harder to be angry if you are both sitting
- think carefully
- be careful with your language: 'It would help me to make a plan if I knew what was on your mind' is better than: 'What am I supposed to do about it!'
- indicate you are sorry for their response and that you are happy to try and find out what has happened and are willing to try to help
- try to elicit any feelings underlying the anger, e.g. hopelessness, despair, chronic pain
- make good eye contact, look away briefly before replying to show you are considering your response, then glance down to allow space for their reply
- attend: lean forward, unfold your arms
- do not interrupt, let them tell the story as it helps to diffuse the anger
- actively listen and check understanding
- ask what their preferred outcome would be
- offer an expression of regret
- say what you are going to do, then do it.

If the angry patient is on the telephone:

- say 'please slow down so I can write this down'
- remain silent, do not give feedback until the anger is vented
- take control back – summarise
- tell them you are not going to continue the conversation and then hang up.

Strategies to reduce aggression in reception areas

Staff should be trained in:

- assertiveness
- customer care

- risk assessment
- de-escalation skills
- breakaway techniques.

Waiting is difficult. We are all busy people and would no doubt prefer to be somewhere else. It is even more difficult when waiting for important test results, if in pain, or if responsible for noisy or disruptive children. It is important for staff to identify, understand and allow for the stresses that arise while waiting to see a doctor or nurse. Crawford, a psychotherapist at the Tavistock Clinic, London, has also noted the importance of looking at any problems in the waiting area as a symptom of wider conflicts in the surgery.[6] There are loyalties, favourites, alliances and allegiances in the relationships between the practice and the patients to consider. Because of this, it is important for provision to be made for all staff to look at the feelings aroused in them by their contact with patients.

Physical constraints

- Keep reception barriers low and accessible – glass screens irritate and inflame.
- Protective screens are counter-productive – use high wide desks to enable personal contact.
- Use soothing colour schemes – pastels and pinks.
- Favour informal arrangements of seating, not rigid lines.
- Colour code patient files to identify those who have difficulty controlling their anger.
- Use furniture that is screwed to the floor.
- Use visual alert systems, alarms, CCTV.
- Involve crime prevention teams.
- Distribute personal alarms.
- Minimise items that may be used as weapons.

Systems

- Have a system for communicating who is in and out of the building.
- Use a diary for all visitors to the building to sign in and out.
- Discourage unarranged visits and start a search after a two-hour buffer zone.
- Ask community staff and lone workers to report back after visits, double up if visiting high risk patients.

Managing your own anger

If you find yourself being overly aggressive, irritable and angry with people, you are obviously stressed, and clearly not coping. Anger is the most seductive of human emotions – a self-righteous monologue propels it along. In a work environment it has to be controlled, for the sake of your own professionalism and sanity, and out of respect for others' feelings. The following points will help you manage it and achieve control:

- count to 10
- do not vent your feelings
- look at the reality
- know the warning signs: heat, wanting to shout, tears, tight chest
- does how you are behaving match with how you want to be seen?
- change your habitual behaviour pattern and reframe your attitude
- monitor your thoughts and words
- practice positive self-talk
- think of new constructive responses
- channel the energy constructively – find your passion against injustice, for example
- employ quick relaxation techniques to relieve the tension and anxiety – inhale deeply, do some isometric exercise
- decrease your volume
- focus on the facts
- remark about the situation not the person.

You can help avoid your own anger by building successful relationships.

- Try to adopt a more relaxed and positive approach to people – greet them regularly by name; take time to develop social relationships with colleagues.
- Be more appreciative and positive in your relationships.
- Don't put people down with expressions like, 'You've got to be kidding', or demean them with such comments as, 'I thought at least you would know better'. Give yourself time to think more thoroughly and fairly about what you're going to say.
- Do not blame others for failing to meet your own ideals. Point out that we should all learn from our mistakes. Don't make faults in others an excuse for your own failures and disappointments.
- Don't be the type who greets every new suggestion or request with a reason why it won't work, or can't be done. Next time someone asks you to do something, respond with a positive or alternative suggestion.
- Be assertive – if somebody incenses you by asking for a long document to be read and commented on at 5 pm on Friday, respond reasonably: 'I can do it tomorrow first thing, at the moment this other job takes priority'.

Or, 'I realise your job is important, but I am leaving the office now so I'll do it first thing on Monday'.
- Make yourself aware of the effect of your behaviour on other people.
- If you think your behaviour is hostile, ask for feedback, and be prepared for frankness!
- Mind your ego.
- Respect life, people and other approaches.
- Be proactive not reactive.
- Focus on commonalities rather than differences.
- Avoid gender-biased attitudes, categorising and generalising.
- Describe instead of interpreting.

Check the motives behind your behaviour:

- Danger signs
  - hurt
  - envy
  - resentment
  - resistance
  - retaliation
- Are you operating according to your principles or in response to theirs?
- What is your intention in the interaction?
- Do you want to manipulate, hurt, teach a lesson, or resolve the issue?

You should look for recurring patterns in your life:

- Who makes you angry?
- What events trigger your anger? Someone not listening to you? (Challenge this – take charge – 'It's important for me to be heard here. My feelings do count'.)
- When and with whom do you feel safe enough to express your anger?
- What are the messages you have heard about anger?
- What happens to your body when you feel angry?
- What physical ways do you have for letting off steam?

References

1   Fred Pryor Seminars (1994) Pryor Resources Inc., Shawnee Mission Parkway, KA.

2   Green DR (2000) The rising tide of complaints. *Pulse*. 15 December.

3   Jennings T (2001) Clinical Casebook: preparing the ground for breaking bad news. *Registrar Pulse*. 30 June, p. 47.

4   James O (1999) Dealing with aggression. *Community Care*. 4–10 March.

5   Braithwaite R (1999) Anger management. *Community Care*. 16–22 September.

6   Crawford N (1990) *The Psychology of Waiting and Reception in the Surgery.* Participant notes from a 1990 Management in Medicine Conference.

Further reading

Griffin J (1999) *Breaking the Cycle of Depression: a revolution in psychology.* The Therapist Ltd, London. www.mindfields.org.uk.

CHAPTER 7

Dealing with criticism

If you are the kind of person who dreads appraisals and takes any criticism, however well meant, very personally, this chapter is for you. It is usual to feel prickly and defensive, or devastated when criticised. These feelings can be overwhelming, preventing a rational, adult response. Of course, an assertive response is only a tool, and although it can be learnt, it does not replace the need for you to investigate the reasons why you respond as you do. It is only through looking at and understanding these reasons, however painful, that we can begin to understand ourselves and respond authentically, not reactively.

Gael Lindenfield, author and assertiveness trainer, said 'Assertive people are not frightened of criticism because they are well prepared for it and know that it can be useful to all parties concerned'. One of the ways to prepare yourself is to know your likely reactions.

- Build up some self-awareness. Once you have an idea of why you are feeling tearful or defensive, you will be more prepared to tolerate these ambiguous or difficult feelings. From this position, you can act more clearly. You will be more able to accept criticism from others, and also be able to give it yourself.
- Learn to distinguish between criticisms which are valid, invalid, or simply a put-down.

Types of criticism

Valid criticisms are those that you know are legitimate. Only you know if you truly are an impatient person, or always late, or change your mind a lot; so if people accuse you of these you know it does apply, and you need to learn to accept the comment graciously rather than getting defensive.

- Learn to listen carefully to what people are saying. There may be times when you need to accept the truth.

- If you cannot accept a criticism instantly, no matter, think about what was said and return to it another time. It may well be that whatever is being said is unpalatable, certainly it may be something about yourself you do not want to hear or accept. Ask yourself if there is some truth in the criticism.
  - Do you have a tendency to bully and to use your position to get what you want at the expense of others?
  - Do you sometimes feel inadequate so you assert yourself unnecessarily and cause others to feel small or powerless as a consequence?
  - Are you judgemental? (It feels easier to criticise and blame others rather than look inside at your own failings and weaknesses?)

If you feel defensive and angry there is probably some truth in what others are saying.

Invalid criticisms are those that you know within yourself to be clearly untrue, and do not have to be accepted:

- they are often global statements or accusations such as: 'You're so mean/ lazy/unsociable'
- if they feel completely unfair and incorrect, then say so
- these comments are more likely to be said in anger, and reflect the other person's feelings more than your own.

Manipulative criticisms lead you to feel 'put down' in some way, someone is trying to score a point using you as the bait.

- These comments are made by people who probably don't feel good about themselves, and need to make others feel bad in order to feel better themselves: (I'm not OK, you're not OK).
- These types of comments look like a compliment or casual comment on the surface, but in fact on reflection are something more unpleasant. They are the veiled comments that make you feel angry or hurt.
- If you confront the person, and venture to say that their comment hurt you, you may be met with denial: 'Oh, I didn't mean it like that!'. They are the kind of remark used to create a reaction.

Below is an example of an effective response to this sort of situation:

Sarah is a practice manager. She has had the decorators in her room for over four days; the place had been in chaos. Work carried on as usual, meetings were held, and visitors were seen, in an area cordoned off for the purpose. It was the end of the fourth day and Sarah was just about to lock up when one of the decorators, who was packing up, turned to her and said:

'Of course I had a run in with one of you lot years ago, trying to get a doctor to see my brother, but it didn't help. I think you managers are all very well but the way the health service is going I reckon they'd be better off spending all that money on doctors and nurses instead of frittering it away on things that don't do much good. Seems to me the money could be better spent on getting those doctors out to see people instead of getting them to push paper all the time. No offence to you, dear, but really, don't you think you'd be better off helping out in reception instead of swanking around up here?'

Sarah could respond by going into a long diatribe or justification for her service; proving to him that any big organisation needs someone to take charge; detailing the chronic under-funding of the health service overall. Instead, she sees this situation for what it is, someone with a personal grudge to bear, and an outsiders' knowledge of the service through the media. She quickly decides that she doesn't want to be drawn into a lengthy, defensive discussion so she says:

'Derek, I know you'd like to chat but I've had a long day and I'm tired. I'm going to lock up now. Do you want to let yourself out?'

She thus understands his need to off-load, but explains how she feels, ignores the bait, and terminates the conversation by asking an unrelated question.

- Put-downs are designed to make you feel small.
- Can be subtly disguised as social niceties or jokes.
- If you respond with sarcasm, it may be viewed as indirect aggression, and is certainly more competitive than constructive.
- Invest your energy in asserting your own needs, or in taking some positive action to get what you want.

In responding to put-downs, experts suggest that you aim to:

- protect your rights and self-esteem
- let the other person know that you recognise the hidden message
- put a quick stop to the put-down behaviour.

How to deal with common put-down lines from your boss

Whenever I've used these lines it is because I've felt tired, stressed, insecure and unsure of my authority and position. Put-downs need dealing with firmly and honestly. Make it the speaker's problem, not yours. Expose the dishonesty, take them at their word:

'If this were up to me, I'd agree to it, but ...'

- Find out who is responsible.
- Tell them your boss has supported you.

- Get more information about the decision maker that you can use in your favour.

'This is a lot more complex than it looks'

- Tease out and deal with the stated complexities.
- Ask for a quick summary of the issues.
- Focus on the key elements.
- Use to develop a common understanding of the issue.

'I don't think there is time to take your ideas on board'

- Ask them to explain why the deadline is so tight.
- Would there ever have been time for your input, and if not, why not?
- Get them to accept your ideas in principle, finding ways to change the time frame.

'If you'd done this yourself you would know'

- Move the issue onto common ground so you can talk in equal terms.
- Acknowledge the feelings: 'I do respect your experience but I'd like to find a way of understanding your perspective on this'.

'I don't think you need worry yourself about this'

- Say you'd find it really valuable if you could understand the finer points.
- Stress how much your understanding can help them.

'There are other agendas you don't know about'

- Establish your legitimate interest in the matter.
- Get that accepted.
- Ask the speaker to be more specific.

Giving criticism

- Allow the other person *time to prepare*; give some indication of the matter you wish to discuss.
- *Act quickly*. If you defer, and wait until the next time the problem arises, your feelings about the issue will, if anything, be stronger, and hence less controllable.
- Set aside time to talk about the issue in a place where you will *not be disturbed*. Give yourself plenty of time to plan what you are going to say beforehand.
- *Be specific*. Instead of dropping vague hints that you are irritated by poor time keepers, confront the issue: 'Helen, we feel frustrated when you are late, could you try and arrive by 4 o'clock next time?'
- Be prepared to *compromise*: 'If this is difficult for you maybe we could all discuss starting the meeting later ...'.

- *Express how you feel* about the behaviour, and the effect it has on you, the organisation or the patients. Take responsibility for your feelings: 'I feel angry and hurt when ...'.
- *Avoid direct attack and blame* whether in the form of 'You're so immature' or 'You should be more ...'. This can be read as unsolicited, unwanted advice. Do not judge. Global or generalised statements about someone's behaviour are basically attacks on their personality. Avoid labels or stereotypes, for example: 'You're such a wimp', 'That's a typical female response'. Again, state how you feel, specifically, about the one item of behaviour you want changed.
- *Do not assume* you know what motivates other people, for you may be mistaken. Avoid analyses such as: 'She must have known how much that would hurt' – it is impossible to interpret other peoples' behaviour.
- *Spell out the consequences.* These may be positive: 'I will feel much less strained if you could be on time' or 'I feel resentful when you leave all the paperwork to me. I know you don't like doing it but I would like to share the load more equally. That would leave me more time for helping on reception'.

If the consequences are negative, spell them out too. Clarity helps people in their decision making. Choose the level you want: 'I would feel much happier if ...' or 'If there is no change, I will have no option but to leave'.

If the change you anticipate or hope for does not come about, be prepared to ride the consequences. Remember that we can always change our behaviour, but we cannot expect others to change theirs, however much we want them to. You can ask, but you may not get what you want.

- View the other person *as an equal.* If you do take the initiative to confront, remember that you in turn may be confronted.
- *Take responsibility.* Invariably, people are surprised, and often shocked, when you mention that part of their behaviour has had such an effect on you; so do take responsibility for not mentioning it before:
  - 'I'm sorry that I didn't make myself clear before'
  - 'I take full blame: you weren't to know'
  - 'I should have mentioned it before, but I didn't feel able'
  - 'I should have sorted it out and been direct but I was frightened of your reaction'.
- *Take the initiative.* Even if you have taken the initiative to confront, use the opportunity to invite criticism: 'I should have mentioned this before, I expect I've surprised/upset/angered you'.
- *Empathise.* Understand the other person's position. Start with something on the lines of: 'I realise that what I have to say will be upsetting ...'.
- *Keep calm.* Make sure that you keep your voice level and avoid using threatening gestures.
- *Phrase positively*: 'It would be better if you talked more loudly' gives someone the hope of being both better heard and better regarded if they make

that change. Saying the same thing negatively 'It would be better if you did not talk so quietly' can leave the person concentrating on their sense of failure rather than wanting to improve.

- *End on a positive note.*

Find a remark to balance the interaction, give some indication that you value the other person and are not only seeing the negative: 'I'm grateful to you for listening' or 'I'm glad that we've aired this'. If you wish, you may like to add a positive statement about the other person: 'I do hope that my having said this will not adversely affect our relationship. I've always found you especially easy to talk to, and I do value the way we work so well together'. Or you may prefer to end the conversation with a positive consequence; something on the lines of: 'I'm glad that we've cleared the air. Now I feel that I'll be more relaxed in your company'. Be honest and true to yourself, mean what you say.

What is your reaction to criticism?

Very few people are truly invulnerable to criticism and most of us would admit to one of the following reactions:

Non-assertive responses

- Do you avoid the person criticising?
- Are you aggressive?

Avoiding behaviour

Do you avoid criticism by:

- keeping quiet
- ingratiating yourself to others
- staying in a position of less authority or responsibility than you are capable of.

This may be a valid option in intolerable circumstances to take yourself out of a difficult situation, but if you regularly avoid confrontation:

- this passive behaviour can irritate others
- it does not do you justice in your ability to deal with life
- it does not enhance self-development
- it becomes easy to accept and absorb the criticism
- avoidance decreases your self-esteem and does not enhance your confidence
- it damages you in the long term by building up anger and resentment.

Assertive behaviour

Here are some examples of how assertiveness experts would recommend you deal with criticism, using the techniques developed by Anne Dickson.[1]

Agree

This is a useful technique to use with hostile or constructive criticism.

- Check if the criticism applies to you.
- If it is valid and legitimate, then thank your critic for the feedback.
- Agree: 'Yes, I am very untidy', 'Yes, I agree, it was stupid of me to respond to him so aggressively'. In agreeing you disarm your critic if they are using the criticism as hostile bait and develop self-acceptance.
- Be honest. If it is a trait you rather like in yourself, say so. If someone criticised you for being a perfectionist you could respond by saying: 'Yes, I am a perfectionist, and I know that sometimes I expect too much from the staff, but I think that it's a good trait and I'm not prepared to lower my standards'.
- If someone criticises you in an area that you are trying to improve, say so: 'Yes, I know I'm being a bit diffident, I'm finding it difficult to make up my mind on this one. I'm sorry if it's a bit irritating, but I am trying to learn to be more concise. I am improving, but I need time'.

Deny it

If the criticism is totally invalid, do not accept it at all, but say with conviction: 'That's completely untrue/unfair/unjust, I am not going to accept that'. Be certain and do not apologise or doubt.

Accept with reservation

Ask for specification if you feel the criticism is global or unjust. This makes it more manageable. If one of your GPs accuses you of *always* being late, and you feel this is untrue, you could say: 'No, I don't accept that I'm always late. I was late today, and I know that I arrived late for that meeting last month, but as a rule I am on time'.

Accept the part of the criticism that is valid, but do not take on board the sort of sweeping generalisation that, if accepted, could gradually lower your self-esteem. Calmly acknowledge that there may be some truth in what is being said. Make your own assessment of the situation: 'Yes I was late this morning. Possibly I am not as committed to work at the moment as I usually am'.

Accepting criticism:

- is very powerful
- reinforces the idea that you alone have the right to act as a judge of your own behaviour
- refuses to reward the critic who is trying to put you down
- acknowledges there is some truth in their statement
- encourages the critic to learn to be more specific with their criticisms.

Ask for examples

Sometimes you feel that a criticism has a grain of truth in it, or you feel uncertain if your critic is manipulating you. This technique:

- gives you time to think
- enables you to hear a little more about what the other person is trying to tell you; if the criticism is constructive you will be able to use that information to learn
- is used to prompt criticism
- because you are initiating it, enables you to operate from a position of strength.

Below are some examples of this:

- 'In what ways do you think I am lazy?'
- 'You say that you are concerned that I am too critical in my dealings with patients. Can you give me some examples?'
- 'Are you saying that you are dissatisfied with the quality of my work?'
- 'Do you find me a bit too pushy at times?'
- 'Are you angry that I'm late?'

When you invite criticism you are opening up a frank and truthful exchange of feelings. This is a powerful way of enabling someone to feel secure enough to express negative feelings to you, and also helps you to feel secure enough to listen to what is being said. Here are some of the examples Anne Dickson uses to illustrate this:[1]

- 'I've been very preoccupied lately. Do you find this frustrating?'
- 'I talk a lot when I'm anxious. Does this irritate you?'
- 'I know I'm inconsistent. Does it drive you up the wall?'

Some advantages of this approach are that:

- when you invite criticism, you are in a much stronger position to handle it
- when you choose when you are going to ask, you are back in control of the situation
- the more often you survive hearing something you don't like about yourself, the easier it will be to deal with criticism

- you begin to be able to use the criticism wisely, to judge for yourself what is said, and use the opportunity to learn.

Much criticism is given out of genuine respect and kindness with the wish to reach out and help, to improve communication and deepen understanding. It can demonstrate someone's clear regard for you.

Checklist for giving criticism

- Set the scene.
- Act quickly.
- Be specific.
- Do not judge.
- Describe your feelings.
- Be aware of the consequences, both negative and positive.
- Take responsibility.
- Ask for feedback.
- Empathise.
- Keep calm.
- Use the broken record technique.
- Phrase positively.
- End on a positive note.

Checklist for receiving criticism

Distinguish between:

Valid –	If valid: agree
Invalid –	If invalid: reject, part accept, deny or ask for more information
Manipulative –	If manipulative: deflect or ignore

See Appendix A for some exercises that will help you deal more constructively with criticism.

Checklist for giving compliments

- Be sincere.
- Be specific.

Checklist for receiving compliments

- Agree.
- Give thanks.
- Do not reject, deny or minimise. Try: 'Thank you' not 'But I laugh like a hyena!'
- Identify backhanders and deal with as invalid criticisms.
- Challenge some of the fixed, negative ideas you have about yourself: if any are negative, swap them for a positive.

Expect and accept compliments graciously. Make a note over a period of one week of how many compliments you have given, taken, or rejected. Over the following weeks, aim to give one extra compliment away each day and note how you felt and how each gesture was received.

Reference

1   Dickson A (1982) *A Woman in Your Own Right*. Quartet Books, London.

Appendix A

Exercise 1

Identify and list some criticisms you have received from:

Parents

Friends

Partners

Children

Employers

Employees

Are these criticisms fair or not?

Exercise 2

Make a column and, on the left, write down five unfair criticisms about yourself. On the right, write down five fair criticisms.

Unfair	Fair
1	
2	
3	
4	
5	

With a partner, pair up and swap lists. Each person reads out items at random from the lists to his or her partner, who has to respond appropriately, e.g.: 'I feel that is an unfair criticism, I will not accept that. Can you give me an example of when I am mean ...' or 'I accept that criticism. I do tend to be bossy, and I'm trying to stop it'.

Exercise 3

With a friend, both write down ten valid criticisms, ten that you consider in-valid (remember you may need to revise these later!) and ten things that you like about yourself. Be specific, so instead of using words like 'good', 'bad' or 'nice' try 'excellent', 'incompetent', 'friendly'. Here is part of my list:

Valid:
- I talk too much.
- I'm too bossy.
- I'm impatient.
- I'm a perfectionist.

Invalid:
- I'm lazy.
- I'm disorganised.
- I'm too critical.
- I'm unsociable.

Personal positives:
- I'm very friendly.
- I'm competent in my job.
- I can put people at their ease.

Swap lists, and then each person randomly reads out items from the list to their partner, beginning with that person's name, e.g. 'Olivia, you're too bossy'. The partner has to respond appropriately, using the skills outlined above, e.g.:

'Yes, I accept that I am bossy. Part of my job is to tell people what to do.'
'I feel that is an unfair criticism. I will not accept that I am disorganised. Can you give me an example?'
'Thank you. I'm proud of the work I do here.' (When given a compliment that you are good at your job.)

Exercise 4. Things I do badly

Take it in turns to say the thing you do most badly, e.g. 'I am very bad at keeping time'. In the next round, each says the thing that other people tell them they do well, e.g. 'People say I'm a good listener'. In the next round, stand up, and tell your partner about the thing that you do well. Ham it up, exaggerate it, and show off: 'I'm the world champion at ...'.

Exercise 5

Look honestly at those aspects of your behaviour that you suspect irritate, disappoint or anger others. Be honest with yourself. Write down those aspects and what you could say to those people if you were to use the skills of negative assertion and negative enquiry.

CHAPTER 8

Negotiating

There are many situations at work when we find ourselves negotiating, either formally or informally. Informal negotiations occur many times a day – whenever we are approached and asked to do something, when one party says 'no' or wishes to redefine or set limits on the activity. Formal negotiations occur on a larger scale – between governments and trade union officials, for example. This chapter identifies the skills and knowledge required to negotiate effectively.

What kind of animal are you?

- *The pigeon*: you're good at your work, liked and respected by all, but don't get promoted.
- *The chameleon*: you've become indistinguishable from the surrounding scenery – you do a good job but nobody knows it.
- *The wild-cat*: when things don't go your way you become aggressive – you are your own worst enemy.
- *The sloth*: you have potential, but somehow never get organised in your work so your ability is never mobilised for your own advancement.
- *The whining watch-dog*: you constantly complain about work demands, the work environment, the way people behave towards you and you're always on the lookout for something to complain about.
- *The willing horse*: smiling sweetly, you say yes to every request.
- *The mule*: for fear of being exploited, you object to every request.

Do you need to learn how to negotiate?

Exercise 1

1   Referring to negotiations that you have been involved in, jot down the factors that helped them to succeed.
2   Note down five points that you think describe negotiating.
3   What are the main differences between negotiating as a team and negotiating as an individual?

A commonly held view is that negotiating means getting your own way. This may not be the case. A better definition may be *discussion producing mutual settlement or compromise*. Negotiation is not about winning at someone else's expense. It is both desirable and necessary that both parties leave the discussion feeling they have gained something. It is about managing, and avoiding, conflict.

There should be movement in both parties – concessions are made only in return for something else. In protracted or formal negotiations both parties could shift or move their position some considerable way.

Preparation

Before embarking on a negotiation:

- choose your objectives and make certain they are realistic. For example, if you want a break from work, would you like an extended holiday, unpaid leave, or a sabbatical? Would it be better to change from full-time to part-time working? Could you arrange a job share?
- look at the results of previous negotiations and what others have been granted in similar positions. For example, is paid study leave the norm in your organisation? Has any other senior member of staff had their hours changed favourably?
- assess your own negotiating power. Look realistically at what you are worth in your job. What is your commitment to the organisation? What does your track record look like?
- understand the other party's plan. What is their position in the hierarchy? What specific limitations are to be expected?
- be aware of the personal and political constraints held by the other party. What will they gain from your plan? Be aware of some of the arguments they are likely to use and prepare your response.

Both parties need to understand the negotiating procedures and the jargon used.

- What is your 'fall back' position? (The least you are prepared to settle for.)
- What 'concessions' are you willing to make? (Those things you are prepared to give up to gain what you want.)
- What are the consequences of withdrawal? You can refuse to continue negotiations if they become unfavourable, but plan a strategic withdrawal rather than just walking out – this may cause you to lose face if the talks are resumed at a later date.
- What is the 'hidden agenda'? Be aware of the undercurrents.
- Prepare a contingency plan if you fail to achieve what you want.
- Choose the right time and place. Avoid a time when the opposition may be under pressure and clarify with them beforehand what you want to discuss so that they also have time to prepare.

Strategies

When preparing to negotiate, work out the strategies to be used beforehand.

- Role play or note them down.
- Avoid using a straight 'no'. There is a need to establish some sort of overlap with the other party because without common ground and understanding, negotiation becomes impossible. Be prepared to move your ground even if only slightly.

It is said there are two main skills used by negotiators: diagnostic and social skills. People with good diagnostic skills are able to probe and analyse, while the basic social skills provide the ability to listen, question, clarify and manage the feelings involved.

You must develop a positive attitude and be aware of distractions used or side issues and irrelevancies thrown up by the other party that may confuse the issue. If this happens, be firm and ask for clarification, or reaffirm the issue in hand:

- use your powers of observation
- summarise often to aid understanding.

During the negotiations:

- try not to use threatening or provocative behaviour
- if you do threaten at any stage, you need to be prepared to follow it through
- find common ground – you want both parties to leave the negotiation feeling successful
- test, understand and summarise

- evaluate
- if in doubt, be prepared to adjourn.

Avoid:

- words with emotive content: 'A generous offer' for example
- spirals of defence and attack
- counter proposals
- position taking.

Successful negotiators explore a wide bargaining range and plot issues sep-arately, breaking items down into smaller units for discussion. Clarification and questioning skills are essential in this procedure. Assertive skills that need to be used are the 'broken record' technique: the need to repeat oneself if the other party goes off at a tangent, has misunderstood, or is using distracting side issues. You need to be able to empathise with the other party, and acknowledge you have understood their position: 'I can see that you are unhappy about it, but I cannot complete the work today; I could finish it by Tuesday though' – state your compromise.

There can be a lot of stress involved in some confrontations, and emotions and feelings run high. Try to remain cool and retain your credibility. Be aware of and be proud of your own skills, and use your knowledge of these in the bargaining procedure.

Both parties should leave the negotiating table feeling happy about the out-come. Guidelines should be established regarding any agreements reached, any follow-ups required, and dates specified for implementation.

Below is an example of tactics to employ when negotiating a pay rise.

Preparation

- Do your homework and familiarise yourself with both the grades and rates of pay.
- Get copies of relevant pay scales as guidelines, with outline job descrip-tions to match suggested grades.
- Check to see if you feel you are being paid unfairly.
- See if there are any areas of work that you currently undertake that are not reflected in your current rate of pay, and any areas you aspire to that you could offer as added value to the practice.

Always ask for more pay if you take on any job that is clearly more substantial in terms of responsibility, e.g. if you are now single-handedly taking respon-sibility for a block of work, where before you worked under supervision. Use the scales and grades as a guideline to support your case.

Before even considering embarking on a negotiation, choose your objectives and make certain they are realistic.

Example 1: The practice manager's agenda

Look at the results of previous negotiations and what others have been granted in similar positions.

- What is the general rate of pay for managers with a practice of your size in your area?
- Look honestly at what you are worth in your job.
- Look honestly at the pay scales.
- What is your commitment to the organisation?
- What does your track record look like?
- What 'extras' can you offer?
- What is your 'fall back' position? (The least you are prepared to settle for.)
- What 'concessions' are you willing to make? More hours for more pay? Reduced holiday?
- Prepare a contingency plan. For example, an ideal settlement might be a 5% increase; a realistic settlement 3% and the fall back position increased holiday.
- What would it feel like to lose? Be prepared for this.

Example 2: The GP's agenda

Be aware of some of the arguments they are likely to use and prepare your response.

- Look at, and understand, the GP's plan: they will not want to pay any more, but they might want to keep you: it may be an awkward time for you to leave – capitalise on this.
- Do they want you to further your role?
- What will they gain from your plan?
- Can they afford you?
- Will they be able to support your claim to the PCT if they want to increase the amount they are being reimbursed?
- What are their present profit levels like? Are they bemoaning the fact they have not had a pay rise in the last three years – if so, it is not a good time to act. Wait until they are more buoyant, or until you have brought a large sum of money into the practice or received outside accolades.

If they don't want to pay you, go for enhanced non-pay items such as increased holiday or enhanced benefits.

Be prepared for the partners to refuse point blank, but it is more likely that they will redefine your terms or set limits: remember to concede some things, they will need to feel they have also gained something from the discussions.

Prior to the negotiation

- Choose the right time and place.
- Avoid a time when the 'opposition' may be under pressure.
- Clarify with them beforehand what you want to discuss so that they also have time to prepare.
- Write a letter outlining your case, and ask to meet the partners to discuss the matter.
- This is a formal negotiation; do not let it be by-passed or undermined as a side issue in another impromptu meeting.
- If necessary, rehearse with sympathetic friends or colleagues.

The negotiation

- Plan for a strategic withdrawal if you need time to think: adjourn.
- What is the 'hidden agenda'? Be aware of the undercurrents.
- Remember it will be unusual if you get your own way entirely.
- You will have a discussion, hopefully producing a mutual settlement or compromise.
- There should be movement in both parties – concessions are made only in return for something else.
- Remember that both parties could shift or move their position some considerable way.
- Both parties need to leave the discussion feeling that they have gained something.
- Avoid personal argument.
- Avoid using a straight 'no': without common ground and understanding, negotiation becomes impossible.

Develop your people skills

- Use good diagnostic skills: probe and analyse.
- Use your basic social skills: listen, question, clarify and manage the feelings involved.
- Develop a positive attitude.
- Be alert to the possibility of distractions.
- Use your powers of observation.
- Summarise often to aid your own understanding.
- Prepare to feel stressed but try to remain cool.
- Retain your credibility.

Tactics

Be clear and specific.

- Make the statement simple, brief and direct.
- Own your statement, assume responsibility.
- Be firm and clear and avoid unnecessary padding.
- Seek clarity from the other party if you are not sure, or feel muddled and unhappy.
- Clarity untangles unexpressed needs or manipulation.
- When you express a willingness to accept the situation and look at changing it, you regain the power.

Be open and honest about your feelings.

- Take personal responsibility for your feelings.
- Begin difficult situations with simple statements, for example: 'I feel nervous ... I know this is difficult for both of us ...'. The immediate effect is to defuse or reduce your anxiety enabling you to relax and take charge of yourself and your feelings.
- Self-disclosure demonstrates that you have a greater acceptance of all the aspects of your personality, which shows greater maturity and professionalism.

Repeat your message.

- Remember the 'broken record' technique: if you feel misheard, calmly repeat your statement or request.
- Maintain your position without being influenced by manipulative comment, irrelevant logic or argumentative bait: the negotiators will accept and respect your clarity, determination and ability to set your own priorities.

Listen and understand, but do not necessarily agree.

- Listen carefully to the other person's point of view, acknowledge it, and then stick to your desired point.
- Do not be led by anyone else's aim to control the agenda. This is your agenda, so avoid any diversion by clever and articulate argument. Stay with what you need, relax and keep to your word.
- Indicate that you have heard what is said; acknowledge the other person's point of view, while still continuing confidently with your request or statement. 'I understand that you are concerned about your own drop in pay over the last year or so, and this is something I am sure you have taken up with the appropriate authorities. My concern is with my pay and conditions of work, and this is what we need to get back to now'.

Demonstrate you are able to understand the other person's point of view, even though you do not necessarily share it.

- There may be attempts to undermine you with criticism: 'But you are never available now when I want to see you, if you did this new work we would never see you'. The request hides frustration and resentment. 'Read' behind the statement, so that your response could begin: 'Yes, I am often absent from the office when you need me. Unfortunately this job does necessitate me being away in meetings fairly frequently, and this will increase as I increase my responsibilities outside the practice. What we need to think about is how I can best meet the practice need to stay in touch – how about more meetings/a mobile/a pager ...'. State your compromise.
- Speak positively about *when* you take on your new role, not *if*.

Prompting others to express themselves

- Seek out criticism about yourself.
- Prompt negative feelings.

This encourages your critics to be more assertive. For example, you may ask: 'Are you finding this difficult to talk about – money always is' or 'Do you think I'm being unfair?'

When behaving assertively, you are confronting issues and situations rather than waiting passively in the hope that you will be able to respond. It is less stressful, and more powerful, to set the agenda yourself.

Accepting criticism

As you take charge of the agenda you communicate more powerfully. You then take the risk of opening the levels of communication. Thus, you must expect honest communication back, including probably some criticism of parts of your work.

- Accept constructive criticism if it is fair or truthful. Examples of your response may be 'yes, I know I can be aggressive at times' and 'you are right, people management is not my best skill. However, we could take this opportunity to build on my strengths and minimise my weaknesses. If I delegate all first line management to X, who is brilliant at it, that would free me up to concentrate on policy and planning'.
- Acknowledge the truth.
- Take up the opportunities offered to change the situation around positively: offer positive alternatives.
- Demonstrate that you remain your own judge.

Empowerment and innovation

Being assertive is a very powerful and freeing tool. Through being assertive you also empower others, allowing them the room to take space and negotiate their needs. As your sensitivity to others increases, so will your ability to feel care, compassion and respect for their agenda.

Some final points about negotiation

- Negotiate from an equal position.
- Be proud of your own skills.
- Never compromise on your self-respect.
- Both parties should leave the negotiating table feeling happy about the outcome.

Having reached an agreement

- Guidelines should be established regarding any agreements reached.
- Check for follow-up.
- Check dates specified for implementation.

Summary of the stages in the negotiating process

- Work out a strategy, remembering timing is very important.
- Decide on objectives, e.g. I want an 8% pay increase; I would like a three week holiday in June.
- Assess your own and others' negotiating power, e.g. What am I worth in my job? What is my commitment to the organisation? My past experience? What is my boss's position in the hierarchy?
- Establish specific objectives:
  - the ideal settlement: 8% increase in pay?
  - a realistic settlement: 5% increase in pay?
  - the fall back position: 4% increase in pay?
- Establish overlap with the other party.

Remember there can be a lot of stress involved in some confrontational situations and emotions run high. Build up your credibility and respond to the others' expectations.

PART TWO

In Part Two we look at how you can apply your developed communication and assertiveness skills to:

- manage time
- manage your own stress levels
- set goals
- manage change
- develop your relationships within your organisation.

CHAPTER 9

Time management

'It's not enough to be busy. The question is: What are we busy about?'

Henry Thoreau

All of us should build rest and relaxation into our working day to keep us sane and effective, but the pace of primary care is such that this is not always possible. Time is a precious resource. Here we identify who and what wastes our time, and some of the ways we can use advanced communication skills to manage these intrusions. GPs, in particular, struggle with time management.

Managing time

If you feel constantly stressed, one key solution is to learn to control events rather than let them control you. Take charge, plan your work, and you will immediately feel less stressed. Proper organisation gives you a sense of direction and control.

When you allow the situation to control you, you are following external and imposed schedules. You then struggle with interruptions, paperwork and procrastination while yearning for freedom and flexibility.

A full working week contains 168 hours, and how you use these is up to you. Some time managers believe that many of us spend as much as 80 per cent of our time on non-essential tasks. There are ways of improving your use of time and so releasing you to do those important tasks.

Time stealing

Time is a finite resource that needs protecting. People who 'steal' time are not usually ill-intentioned. Their demands on you may inadvertently waste your time; they may talk about situations or events unconnected with you, or they may distract you with an activity that may be welcomed at a different time, such as gossip. Team working is dependent on good relationships, and these good relationships do take time to foster and develop, but the key to managing your time is to be in charge of it. It is up to you to decide, or negotiate, when and where such conversations take place.[1]

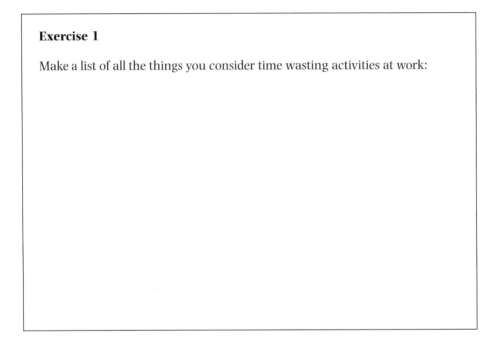

Exercise 1

Make a list of all the things you consider time wasting activities at work:

Here are some ideas that will help you take better control of your time.

Interruptions

Give clear messages to those who interrupt. Your time is expensive.

- Give people who offer you information a chance to indicate if it is urgently important; schedule in a good time to hear it. If not, offer a choice: 'I can only spare about a minute now – can it wait?'.
- Develop 'screening' plans:
  - insist on appointments
  - decide in which situations staff may interrupt you and which things can be postponed
  - then work quietly in your room with the door shut and the phone diverted
  - designate an amount of time each day during which employees agree not to interrupt each other. Use a flag system on the desk: red for 'Do not disturb', orange for 'Come in, but it had better be important', green for availability.

- Use body language: remain standing while you talk, and usher the speaker out by opening the door to indicate their exit.
- Make it clear that the visit/meeting is over, 'Before we finish, I would ...'.
- Tell people at the beginning of the meeting how much time you've allocated to it.
- Stand up when people enter your room. To protect yourself further don't keep a chair near your desk. Both of you will be more likely to stay on target.
- Meet people at *their* desks when you need something from them. By doing this you are in control of the visit and it is easier for you to exit.
- If you feel you are going to ramble, schedule your meetings before appointments.
- To save on travelling time, try to have all meetings in your own office.

Telephones

- Always identify self, department and organisation when answering.
- Have a pen and paper by all phones.
- Don't be kept waiting with an engaged tone – get them to call you back or use a hands-free phone.
- Plan ahead. List items you want to discuss. It saves time for everybody and makes for better communication.
- Create telephone protocols so that everyone can take appropriate responsibility for messages.
- Never let yourself be interrupted from the task at hand by a ringing phone: when you take the calls as they come you allow your work to be randomly disrupted.
- Buy a three-minute sandglass and put it by your phone. See if you can successfully complete every call in three minutes.
- Arrange with co-workers to sign up for certain hours during which one of you will answer the phone for everyone. This gives everyone a bit of protected time.
- Ring people instead of writing them letters, telephone conference instead of meeting. Use e-mail in preference to the telephone.
- Use the phone to inform, not chat.
- Prioritise. Use your secretary/operator/voice mail to screen calls.

Computer

- Utilise all short cuts: use your address books and create easy access systems for numbers/sites used regularly.
- Ask to be notified by e-mail about meetings.
- Use a computerised diary where possible so that everybody can view, but not edit. This reduces the need for some paperwork and memos.

Report writing

- Know the reader and purpose.
- Use the four-step method (prepare, arrange, write, revise).
- Keep it simple.
- Turn weekly reports into monthly reports and monthly reports into quarterly reports.

Crisis management

- Learn to say no! Do one job at a time.
- Ignore the problems which are of minor importance. Delegate those that your subordinates can handle.
- Drop old responsibilities when you accept new ones.

Paper chain

Common irritants in general practice are:[2]

- lost papers
- illegible cryptic scrawls
- incorrect or incomplete facts
- delays in processing paperwork
- failure to follow agreed practice systems or protocols.

Each time a task is not properly completed, the next person involved in the work has an additional burden. Ultimately, all the paperwork in primary care relates to patient care and while one member of the practice may sometimes be indifferent, others are not and they may feel compelled to complete the work properly so that the patient does not suffer.

It should be the responsibility of everybody working in the practice – including the doctors – to ensure that their part of the chain of work is completed in a proper and timely fashion:

- No short-cuts – if these are possible, the system is plainly wrong.
- No putting on one side and forgetting.
- No bucking the system – it was put in place for a reason.
- All staff and doctors should be able to expect others to turn round the paperwork reliably, legibly and accurately.
- Do you tolerate some doctors being disorganised in your practice? Why? In the commercial world and other public sectors it is expected that people must be organised and look after important papers.
- Manage GPs so staff receive a consistent response and behaviour from each one.

- If you are a manager, act like one. Never take on reception or secretarial duties – this is a waste of your time. Discourage other highly skilled and highly paid people within the practice from doing jobs that someone less qualified can do for less.
- Introduce systems: note tracing, message taking and appointments.
- Improve communication, become better organised, and keep the practice clean and tidy. A messy and untidy workplace is disruptive and inefficient. People will have to disrupt each other to ask where things are.
- Use protocols to prevent nurses interrupting doctors, doctors interrupting other doctors and doctors interrupting nurses.

Paperwork

- Avoid scraps of paper for making notes.
- How often do you handle paper? Put a small dot in the upper corner of each piece every time you pick it up to read.
- Analyse *why* you avoid processing some paperwork. Does it bore you or is it difficult?
- Don't be responsible for cluttering up other people's desks.
- Handle each piece of paper once and then act, file, shred or bin.
- If action is required, write notes in the margin, in pencil, with a clear short sentence.
- Annotate as it passes round the practice, with each person initialling their contribution, If a deadline is clearly marked on a letter, ask everyone to add the date they dealt with it. (This not only instils a sense of urgency but also highlights who is sitting on letters and who is dealing with them promptly.)
- Designate one of the lower drawers of your desk as a 'dump' drawer. Into this drawer will go all low-priority items such as routine reports, brochures, newspaper cuttings and other pieces, which aren't urgent. Let these items ripen for a month then *dump* them.
- Have only one item you're working on in view at a time.
- Keep a file to remind you of forthcoming deadlines, important things to do and projects to follow up. This has two major divisions; the first is a set of 12 file folders (one for each month of the year), and the second is *one* set of folders for each day of the month. The current month is placed first in the drawer with the days behind it. Prioritise them.
- Date stamp all documents arriving in the practice.
- Use a post book: record all incoming and outgoing mail.
- Leave letters unsealed until the post is ready to be franked and posted so the sender can retrieve or add to the contents.
- Throw away circulars from outside agencies about things you cannot influence and which do not affect your working life.

- Immediately delete junk e-mails and faxes.
- Sort correspondence into a logical priority order.
- Delegate the routine correspondence to others.

Speed reading

- Preview each section before you read, then read and relate the details to the overall theme. This strategy improves your comprehension and recall.
- Take a moment to practise this on a book. With your hand in a relaxed position, sweep it down the middle of the pages. Do not go all the way to either margin, but stop about a quarter of an inch short of the print on each side of the page. Allow the movement of your hand to guide your eyes smoothly down the page. Do not force your eyes to follow your hand exactly; instead let them drift back and forth looking for ideas.
- Allocate a specific time for reading: use the daytime to meet people and the early morning and evening to read.
- Swap reading. Arrange for a colleague to read certain articles or journals and you read others. Lunch together regularly to exchange information and cuttings.
- Recognise that more can be less. Ominous looking volumes often aren't as long as they appear. Only read what you need to in order to understand the main point.

Delegate

Delegate anything someone can do *better*, *quicker*, *cheaper* than or *instead* of, you. But not:

- confidential matters
- legally/contractually restricted jobs
- disciplinary actions
- ultimate accountability.

Why is it so hard to delegate?

Although it is relatively easy to get people to agree that delegation is worthwhile, many do not delegate as effectively as they could. There are reasons for this, find which one is familiar to you:

- you manage your own time badly, you are overstretched and spend time doing instead of planning
- your responsibilities and limit of authority are not clear to you, or anyone else in the practice

- you under-estimate the competence of your subordinates and genuinely believe that you can do the work better than anyone else
- you feel threatened by the competence of your subordinates
- you feel insecure in your job and in your work relationships.

Learn how to delegate, not abdicate. Delegation is crucial in any place of work. Doctors, chief executives, directors, managers and supervisors all have a responsibility to delegate some of their work so that they can concentrate on those tasks that only they are best able, and are paid, to do. It is very common in general practice to find poor patterns of delegation: it is an underused art.

See the author's book, *Communication and the Manager's Job*, for more information on managing meetings and delegation.[3]

Management of meetings

Here are some facts about meetings in general practice:

- most people don't like meetings
- meetings are essential to foster good two-way communication
- meetings need to be held regularly
- partners demonstrate their commitment to their employees through attending meetings
- practices must feed back to the staff following meetings where staff have been excluded
- staff need to feel included in the major decision making.

Note if your meetings are well chaired, well organised or not, have good attendance, are held frequently enough, or if there is an absence of agendas and minutes.

Well planned and managed meetings are an organisation's most valuable means of communication – they considerably ease the task of coordinating the activities of large and diverse organisations like the health service. *See* Appendix A for a questionnaire on how effectively you manage your meetings.

Problem meetings

Dr Vivien Martin discusses some common themes to managing unproductive meetings, which she attributes to ineffective control of people and time.[4] Here are some suggestions.

- The chair must demonstrate control of the meeting.
- Interrupt and move unproductive time wasters or hecklers on to something else.

- Summarise and restate if people are inarticulate or rambling, or simply glance obtrusively at your watch.
- Manage personality clashes as these can factionalise your group and severely hamper discussion:
  - draw attention back to the point of the meeting
  - cut across the argument with direct questions on the topic
  - restate group boundaries: 'We need to keep personalities and judgements out of the discussion'
  - reiterate the objective of the discussion and the time pressures on the meeting
  - point out the constraints under which everyone is operating
  - suggest that they discuss the problem with you privately or raise the issue in a more appropriate forum.

Meetings need to be tightly managed

- Prevent side conversation.
- Meetings often contract (or expand) to fill the time allotted. Shorten them.
- Give incentives to stay on target: meet before lunch or late afternoon.
- Review the frequency and duration.
- Use definite times/meetings for discussing routine matters with others.
- Start and finish on time, and never relay the meeting for latecomers.
- Postpone or delegate topics that need further discussion or research.
- Produce action minutes with name and deadline.
- Only speak if you have a real contribution to make.
- Avoid all meetings that do not run smoothly.
- Delegate housekeeping responsibilities.
- Use a skilled, firm and authoritative chair. Interrupt people who:
  - begin philosophical discussions
  - tell long-winded jokes or anecdotes
  - rehearse or re-play meetings without reference to the agenda or minutes.
- Ask 'why are we meeting?' If an agenda cannot be produced, there is no meeting.

Deal with lateness[5]

- *Calculate the cost of lateness.* If you have 20 people attending a meeting which starts ten minutes late, your organisation has lost the equivalent of half a day's work.
- *Interrupt lateness*: it shows a strong contempt for people and lack of respect for their time. Bad timekeepers are usually bad administrators – poor

at making decisions, unable to say no, incapable of critical path analysis, and bad at setting priorities. Try to establish a sharper routine.

- *Be prompt.* If you let meetings begin late, you are penalising those who have arrived promptly. Never recap for latecomers, but if desperate, start meetings with the least important item. Try to deal separately with latecomers. Give space for punctual colleagues to air their opinion: 'Would anyone like to comment on our timing? Some people were unfortunately delayed – but is there a way we can synchronise our timing better in future?'
- Don't ever keep people waiting as a way of showing how important you are. This could backfire.

How do you spend your time?

If individuals wish to improve their time management then the starting point is to establish how time is currently used. Keeping a 'time diary' can be useful in clarifying not only *how* you spend your time, but also in identifying *who* influences your use of time.

Exercise 2

1   Using the following form, record everything you do at work for 2–3 days. Every minute should be accounted for and you should be as honest as possible. Make a note of each and every time you change your activity – do not leave it until the end of the day – memory distorts time.

2   Record:

- the time
- the activity
- who initiated the activity (yourself, your staff, a patient, a colleague, external colleagues, etc.)
- time taken
- any interruptions (if these are time-consuming they would become activities in their own right).

DAILY TIME LOG AND ANALYSIS

Sheet no _____   Today's priorities:

Name _____   1 _____

Day & date _____   2 _____

                                                          3 _____

Time of day	Activity	Who initiated?	Time taken (mins)	Interruptions	Critical comment

Time worked: _____ hours _____ minutes

Keep a diary record of:
(a) content of work
(b) contacts
(c) work priorities
(d) vital tasks

Set a meeting with yourself at the end of the day to review your daily objectives and set future ones.

Exercise 3

TIME WASTERS' ANALYSIS

Time wasters	Log the time you spend on each time waster							
	Mon	Tue	Wed	Thu	Fri	Sat	Sun	Total
Unexpected visitors								
Inability to say 'no'								
Trying to do too much at once, and under-estimating time required to do the task								
Telephone interruptions								
Coffee/tea breaks								
Personal disorganisation								
Indecision on what to do								
Fatigue								
Crisis situations for which no plans were possible								
Wrong information given about meeting place, etc.								
Surfing the net, etc.								

ELIMINATE TIME WASTERS

Time wasters	Possible causes	Solutions	How you will apply the solutions

---

Exercise 4

List your priorities in terms of work and personal life, giving each a set of goals that you would like to achieve and strategies for achieving them. For example:

Monday
- Write up report.
- Set up meeting with C.
- Send invoices to accounts department.
- Phone GP.
- Write and distribute agenda re: PM.
- Arrange lunch with X.
- Check Y ordered new stationery.

If you find that your activity in the morning is to make all your phone calls, so that by lunchtime you haven't even considered the report, then face it, your strategy isn't working. Ask yourself why and vow in future to concentrate first on the two priority items, before dealing with the remainder, in order.

Don't make the mistake of working so hard to meet your goals that your life becomes imbalanced, or impose too much routine in your daily schedule so that it becomes monotonous. Research has shown that the maximum time anybody should work in a week for ultimate effectiveness is between 35 and 45 hours. Every hour worked over 45 is only about 25% effective in terms of productivity.

See Appendix A for some more time management tips.

Be assertive

Do you passively accept poor delegation, incomplete instructions, too many projects at a time or unclear deadlines? Success at working less and accomplishing more depends on knowing what *not* to do. Over-commitment is one of the most frequent ways we dilute our effectiveness.

- Be selective. Learn to say *no*. Never say yes when you know you could be putting that time to better use.
- Ask, 'Am I the right person for this task?'.
- Do not procrastinate. Answers such as 'I don't know' or 'let me think about it' only raise false hopes. You have the right to say no, and you don't have to offer a reason every time.
- Clarify how much authority you have on assignments, then you can continue without constant approval.

- Repeat directions in your own words so you both are certain you've understood the assignment correctly.

Urgency v importance

- Fixing a flat tyre when you are late for an appointment is a matter of great urgency, but its importance is, in most cases, relatively small. Many of us spend our lives fixing flat tyres and ignoring less urgent but more important matters.
- In many situations, 20% of what you do yields 80% of your results. Concentrate on those high-payoff items. Of the remaining items, ask yourself, 'What is the least work I can do on these and for them still to be acceptable?' Then determine which activities you can delegate, which require your limited thought, and which demand your careful attention.
- When you are faced with a number of problems, ask yourself which are the truly important ones, and make them your first priority. If you allow yourself to be governed by what's urgent, your life will be one crisis after another. A few foresight-taking steps to prevent potential problems may ensure that you spend your time achieving your goals rather than reacting to crises.

Negative emotions

Of all the emotions over not getting more done, guilt is one of the most useless. Regret, remorse and bad feeling can't change the past and they make it difficult to get anything done in the present. Worry, which is future-oriented, is another useless emotion.

Get worry out of your life

- Consider what Mark Twain once said, 'I have known a great many troubles, but most of them never happened'.
- Confront your concern head on. Ask yourself 'What's the *worst* that could come from this?'. When you answer that question, the need for worry usually vanishes.
- Replace negative thought patterns: Replace 'What if X happens?' with 'If X happens I will deal with it by Y'.
- If you imagine a catastrophic event, say to yourself: 'And *then* I would (do X) ...' .
- Replace worrying with action planning. Set yourself meaningful goals and go after them. You'll soon get so absorbed in their pursuit that you won't have time for worrying.

Ridding yourself of negative emotions can make you a new person. You will find you have time, energy and abilities you never dreamed you had.

It is said there is no such thing as time management, as time cannot be managed. But there is self-management. Time does not waste itself, it needs help. Most of us work hard in order to reap the benefits life has to offer. Consider how you can get the greatest return on your investment of time and energy. Strive to work less and accomplish more, but do not demand perfection from yourself. There will never be enough time for everything. But you can do a little less a little better.

References

1   Wynne-Jones M (2001) Time stealers. *Pulse*. 21 April.

2   Hawksley N (2000) Paper chase. *Practice Manager*. August, pp. 21–2.

3   Phillips A (2002) *Communication and the Manager's Job*. Radcliffe Medical Press, Oxford.

4   Martin V (2001) Meetings management. *Practice Manager*. December/January.

5   MacErlean N (2001) How to cope with late colleagues. *The Observer*. 19 August.

Further reading

Adair J (1988) *Effective Time Management*. Pan, London.

De Mare G and Summerfield J (1983) *101 Ways to Protect Your Job*. McGraw Hill, London.

Leboeuf M (1979) *Working Smart*. McGraw-Hill, Maidenhead.

Turla PA and Hawkins KL (1983) Time stretch. *Company Magazine*. November, pp. 64–5.

Appendix A

More time management tips

- Avoid taking work home unless you are certain you will do it, better still, stay half an hour extra and finish the job, and give the evening to your family.
- Do jobs requiring mental effort when you are at your best. You may find that in the morning your ideas are good, but you have trouble getting them on paper; and early afternoon is your period of highest writing productivity. So think about the topics you want to cover in the morning, then jot down ideas and put them aside until early afternoon, when you write them out fully.
- Set up a fixed daily routine. Schedule definite times for routine matters such as meetings, going through the mail, communicating with your secretary, signing letters, etc.
- Fix deadlines for all jobs and stick to them.
- Do not postpone important matters that are unpleasant. They will block your thoughts and reduce your creativity and working capacity. Tasks rarely get more pleasant by being postponed.
- Put off everything that is not important. Many problems solve themselves if you ignore them for a while.
- Hold meetings with yourself. Put a 'please do not disturb' sign on your door, with a note showing when you are available. Ask your secretary or a colleague to take care of any visitors or telephone calls. Tell the others in the practice which time of the day you are not available and tell them exactly when they can get hold of you again. And be there.
- Do one thing at a time. Keep an overview of the next jobs.
- Collect all your ideas in one place. Write down the ideas the moment you get them. Go through your ideas regularly and act on them.
- When you start a piece of work, finish it. If you split it up too much, you lose track of its coherence, lose your overview and waste your time warming up each time you start again.
- Arrange your breaks at times when you cannot work effectively. For instance when the people you have to talk with are not available, when the material you need is not ready, etc.
- Don't do it if you can delegate or ignore it.
- Categorise tasks as important or unimportant, urgent or non-urgent:
  - simple, short-term tasks
  - simple, long-term tasks
  - complex, short-term tasks
  - complex, long-term tasks

Then do them in the following order:

	Important	Unimportant
Urgent	Do first	Delegate
Non-urgent	Do next	Ignore

Plan your day

- Get in the habit of writing a 'to do' list every day.
- Be realistic and aware of the limitations of your time: you can fit in only so many activities. You'll feel much better when you finish 10/10 instead of 10/20.
- Plan for the unexpected such as people being a bit late for appointments.
- To save on travelling time, try to have all meetings in your own office, and if on a tight schedule tell people at the beginning of the meeting how much time you've allocated to it.

Organise yourself

- Tell yourself that you'll work for just ten minutes. After that, you may have begun to get some sort of a momentum and won't want to stop. If you do stop for some reason, you'll be ten minutes closer to your goal.
- Make it a game to finish in time. Cut off your escape. Put away tempting directions.
- Work to natural stopping places. You'll feel less scattered and more satisfied. For example, don't stop reading in the middle of a section. Finish fully.
- If it is your responsibility, deal with big problems yourself immediately, instead of waiting for somebody else to sort it out.
- Start, no matter what, *start*! If you have a phone call to make, pick up the receiver and start dialling. If you have a letter to write, start typing.
- Put time committed to routine daily essentials to a second use: record lecture notes and play them back while dressing or driving to work, use waiting time to plan your weekend, pay bills or write letters.
- Master the art of deskmanship. Many of us perform some or all of our work at a desk. A desk is a tool that aids in the processing of information, *not* a place to collect waste paper, a storage depot for non-job sundries, or a flat surface on which to stack items you want to remember. One time management consultant kept a close time log on an executive with a

stacked desk and found that he spent an average of two hours and 19 minutes per day looking for information on the top of his desk.

Summary

- Get organised.
- Plan your day.
- Clarify objectives.
- Group tasks.
- Do not procrastinate.
- Break up tasks.
- Always have something to read with you.
- Do difficult tasks when you are fresh, routine when less so.
- Avoid perfectionism.
- Reduce interruptions.
- Learn to say no.
- Reward yourself.

CHAPTER 10

Combating stress

Many successful people are approaching 'burn out'. The symptoms of this are reversible. This chapter will assist you to recognise the signs and symptoms of stress, and give you some strategies for dealing with it. We look at what stress is and some of the common causes. Within the appendices are some practical guidelines for managing stress – how you can help yourself and involve other people to assist you.

Signs of stress

Anyone working in health or social care understands stress. In May 2000, a news item in *Practice Manager* reported that:[1]

- practice administration and dealing with GPs are the strongest predictors of practice managers being classified as stressed or depressed
- a total of 82% say they work more than their contracted hours per week
- overtime ranges from one to 18 hours
- the two most common stress-inducing activities are finding locums (50%) and future planning (48%).

The pressures in healthcare are growing relentlessly and remorselessly. Consider the list below. Do you:

- feel guilty when relaxing?
- feel irritable, impatient, frustrated?
- have difficulty concentrating, worry continually?
- feel endlessly tired or suffer from niggling physical complaints?
- feel disorientated when the day's work finishes?
- feel increasingly cynical and disenchanted with your work?
- feel emotionally exhausted, and increasingly forgetful?
- are working harder and harder and accomplishing less and less?
- depersonalise: treat patients as impersonal objects?
- feel you are not achieving as well as you were?

How often do you experience these emotions? How often do you talk about them? If your answer is often, you may be suffering from some of the physical effects of stress, i.e. your muscles feel knotted and tense; you may be smoking or drinking more than usual; you may experience a dry mouth, sweaty palms or an upset stomach in difficult situations. Work may seem full of crises that you never seem to solve; you may lie awake at night thinking, yet be unable to make decisions.

Current estimates are that up to 30% of all GP consultations are stress related. Unpublished medical opinion considers that to be a conservative estimate, and cites that possibly up to 80% of all diseases have psychosomatic origins. Other estimates show high levels of burnout among inner-city GPs in particular, with 44% feeling drained and exhausted and 42% depersonalising patients.[2] Younger GPs seem particularly vulnerable.

There is no doubt that we *could* be happier, healthier and be more productive at work, if stress free. Medical problems are not inevitable and there are many techniques to assist. Most of us will feel that some of the statements above apply some of the time. Indeed, stress needs to be part of everyday life as:

- it helps to keep us alert and out of danger
- in small doses, it can create a 'high' where challenges are enjoyed
- it accounts for feelings of excitement and optimism when a new venture is started.

Any new life event or change does create stress, but we often feel the positive rather than the negative changes. We experience the same physical and mental alertness when we are about to embark on a physically demanding venture, such as preparing for a sporting event, and it is clear that in these circumstances a degree of stress is essential.

- What is stress?
- How can it be important?
- Why does it sometimes 'tip over' to an unwelcome extreme?

Physiological reactions to stress

In a potentially dangerous or threatening situation, our bodies automatically react:

- senses sharpen
- adrenalin, the 'flight or fight' hormone, floods into our bloodstream
- we breathe more deeply and increase our heart rate
- muscles tense in anticipation
- we prepare for action.

Instincts have primed us for self-survival in a classic stress response. However, this bodily preparation is often unnecessary. Our bodies are primed to expect physical attack, and the physical responses experienced are a legacy from a time when we had to fight for our own lives. It takes a good while for the body to return to a calm equilibrium.

Our bodies cannot tell the difference between events that are actual threats to survival and events that are present in thoughts alone. As our society has developed, we have invented situations that are impossible to deal with physically, for instance we cannot escape from a traffic jam and we cannot satisfactorily verbally abuse a computer when it makes an error. We are simply stuck with the feelings and the exaggerated bodily reactions.

Stress, whether acute or chronic, releases a whole array of hormones that provide quick energy. Two of these, adrenalin and cortisol, are potent inhibitors of the immune system. Other changes that occur are:

- the heart rate increases, with a concomitant increase in blood pressure
- our internal organs cease to work effectively as blood flow to them is reduced
- the chemical build-up in our muscles does not dissipate easily and small nodules appear, classically around the neck and shoulder area
- frequent surges of blood pressure can lead to heart disease and stomach tensions can lead to ulcers
- the hormonal residue can cause irritation, frustration, impatience and mood swings.

Because of these changes we then overeat to soothe ourselves, take drugs to ease the upset stomach and use tobacco, drugs or alcohol to artificially calm or deaden the experience.

Causes of stress

List your own causes and begin to develop your self-awareness.

Write down your personal stress triggers

See Appendix A for a table which enables you to identify your personal stress levels.

Our workplace environment and conditions can contribute to stress. Mark off which of these factors are contributing to your stress:[3]

Workplace environment

- Poor light levels and air quality.
- Unmanaged interruptions.
- Infrequent breaks.
- Lack of privacy.
- Low resources.
- Staff shortfalls.
- Essential travel.

The work

- Does everyone understand the nature of your work?
- Do you have a work overload or underload?
- Are you adequately trained for the job?
- Are there any specific demands made of you that are unusual?
- Are your work boundaries defined or vague?
- Is there enough variety in your work?
- Is your work developing?

Relationships

- Are you well managed?
- Do you have good relationships with your colleagues?

Rewards

- Are you paid adequately for the job?
- Are you appraised?
- Is your work acknowledged?

Organisational culture

- What are the expected behaviours in your organisation and do you fit in?
- What is the extent of communication and consultation?
- Are there any internal power struggles?
- Office politics?
- Conflicts with values?
- Is change imposed or managed?

- Are there frequent structural changes?
- Are new technologies and skills being introduced?

Career development

- Promotion prospects?
- Redundancy?
- Retirement looming?
- Training opportunities?

Some of the most common forms of *stress* at work have been identified:[4]

- Intrinsic to the job – working conditions.
- Role in the organisation – underload or overload.
- Relationships at work – especially with the boss.
- Career development – especially mid-life.
- Organisational structure and climate – rules and regulations.
- Home work interface – especially the growth of dual career families.

Personalities and stress

Those working in the public sector have the additional strain of anticipating unwelcome or unknown changes in their job environment with every new change of government. Managers and clinicians have different stresses; both experience lack of time and work overload, have to balance loyalties and are sandwiched between demands from the government, PCT, doctors, staff and patients. This is an uncomfortable position and we fear voicing our disquiet. One manager describes her dilemma:

> 'I can't risk voicing my dissatisfaction to the partners as I want to appear in control. I am ambitious, so I need to keep the status quo. Sometimes I feel that I am fighting a silent battle within myself; I lie awake and think about work at night and feel as though I am being pushed further and further into a corner of my own making.'

Stress is exacerbated when we have a taste of power but cannot wield much influence. Having severe financial or partnership problems creates additional mental and emotional strains; relationships become fraught and easily break down, which creates a new cycle of problems.

Another list reads very differently. This example shows someone trying to tackle his problems constructively – he has got as far as listing his personal stresses at home and at work. From there he hopes to see if a pattern emerges.

> 'There must be something on my list that I can work on immediately, I suppose that I am a "Type A" personality; the sort you might call a high achiever. I enjoy a challenge and am industrious.'

He has identified that there are some things that he likes doing that cause him some degree of stress. This is to be expected – life and living are stressful. One of the ways that he could reduce his stress levels is by managing his time more effectively. The other is to look at those areas of his life that cannot be so easily changed, and change his attitudes towards them.

Here is the part of his list that focuses on work.

1   Time wasters.
2   The telephone.
3   Having projects interfered with.
4   Partner B.
5   Overrunning meetings.
6   Constant interruptions.
7   The future and uncertainty if I change my job.

Once a list is broken down into manageable portions, it is easier to identify a problem and put things into perspective.

- What can you give up?
- What can you change easily?
- What do you need help with?

Identify the areas that feel uncontrollable and discuss this with a mentor; there are some things that we cannot control – like the future – and although this cannot be altered, attitudes can, and it is this area that we shall examine next. We need to believe in our own power, and believe we can get our future exactly how we want it.

Consider these stress-loaded beliefs that many of us hold about ourselves, question their validity, and reframe them constructively (*see* Appendix D).[5]

- I must be loved or liked by everyone, people should love me.
- I must be perfect in all I do.
- All the people with whom I work or live must be perfect.
- I have little control over what happens to me.
- It is easier to avoid facing difficulties than to deal with them.
- Disagreement and conflict are a disaster and must be avoided at all costs.
- People, including me, do not change.
- Some people are always good, others bad.
- The world should be perfect and it is terrible that it is not.
- People are fragile and need to be protected from the truth.
- Other people exist to make us happy and we cannot be happy unless they do so.
- Crises are invariably and entirely destructive and no good can come of them.
- Somewhere is the perfect job, the perfect solution and perfect partner, and all we need to do is search for them.

- We should not have problems. If we do it indicates we are incompetent.
- There is only one way – the true way.

The above list is more relevant for the passive individual, but if you are a hard-driving, aggressive, assertive individual you will have your own problems: you're sometimes ruthless, but more often than not you're praised and rewarded for your activities:

- you take advantage of every opportunity
- push yourself to the limit
- treat tasks unnecessarily as emergencies
- feel guilty when relaxing
- are easily bored
- you are competitive
- high-achieving
- impatient and ambitious for success
- always seek approval from others
- you believe that success comes from doing things at the fastest possible rate.

These 'Type A' personalities tend to work in fast-moving jobs that require an extrovert personality and also quick decision making – they may choose to manage in an environment of rapid change and development.[6,7]
    'Type A' attributes can also be destructive.

- The struggle to achieve more in less time is often at the expense of others, and even your own health.
- These personalities are three times more likely to have coronary heart disease or other stress-related illnesses (breast cancer, colitis, some forms of diabetes, hormonal and sexual problems) than those with moderate, or Type B, personalities.
- Behavioural characteristics include:
    - walking and eating rapidly
    - trying to do two or more things at the same time
    - not allowing for unforeseen events
    - trying to hurry people's speech/finishing their sentences
    - treating people as rivals/competitors rather than friends or colleagues
    - subject to nervous tics or gestures, e.g. incessantly running fingers through your hair.

What can be done to avoid stress?

See Appendix B for a questionnaire to identify how vulnerable you are to stress. There are many ways in which we can deal with stress. Some are preventative, and some actually tackle the feelings at source. The key thing is to try and modify your behaviour.

Behavioural changes

- Develop resilience and inner strength.
- Keep up to date.
- Make sure you are in the right job.
- Create a good team around you.
- Book frequent breaks.
- Develop other interests.
- Be clear you can't do everything.
- Stay psychologically and emotionally fit.
- See a counsellor for support.

Moderate your stress

You can't change your behaviour totally, but you can at least manage it better by moderating your own self-induced stress:

- get organised
- control any behaviour that you recognise as being obsessional or time-dominated
- don't set unrealistic deadlines
- learn to differentiate between urgent tasks and less important aspects of your work
- not everything requires immediate action. Much more important is the quality of the results
- try to restrain yourself from having to be the centre of attention by constantly talking: force yourself to really listen to others
- avoid being too work orientated
- schedule some non-competitive activities into your leisure time. Do not take up a competitive sport like squash – trying to beat an opponent is just as bad in stress terms as trying to beat a work colleague
- learn to enjoy things rather than treating them simply as a means to an end
- learn to laugh more, be lighter on yourself
- in any discussion don't be on the offensive – you're out to talk, not to do battle. Use a balance of logic, assertiveness and good humour.

These cognitive and behavioural changes can help to reduce your stress levels. When pressures are allowed to get out of hand you become less able to deal efficiently with the problems that face you. Take yourself away from the problem and then you can deal with it.

You can also reduce the harmful effects of work stress, and protect yourself against future pressures, by establishing an anti-stress lifestyle. Exercise, relaxation and eating properly will more than repay the time they take. Exercise, for example, counteracts the effects of stress by increasing the levels of endorphins, and categorically improves mental and physical health. In addition to the cognitive recommendations, try the following suggestions.

- Exercise regularly to counteract the increased muscular tensions.
- Food has an important role to play in fighting stress. Surprisingly, how you eat is more important than what you eat when you're under stress. Look at how, what and when you eat. Eat slowly and well. Savour your food.
- If you are under a great deal of stress or emotional trauma, you are likely to need more of the B-complex vitamins, vitamin C and minerals such as zinc. This also applies to people who smoke, drink alcohol or take antibiotics.
- Avoid using *stimulants* such as alcohol, coffee or cigarettes. These exacerbate by artificially altering your physiological balance:
  - alcohol is a sedative, not a stimulant. It dulls the memory and concentration, and impairs performance. Mood swings and emotional outbursts are more common among drinkers
  - if you are getting heavy hints from friends or relatives, and you can't cut down, consult your GP.
- Women are more likely than men to smoke for negative reasons, believing it helps to combat anger and anxiety. Initially, the effects are helpful; a craving that is much stronger than the original stress follows them. Keep on trying to give up. The more you disrupt your habit, the easier it becomes to kick it.
- When you're under stress, relaxation often requires a conscious effort. Develop reflective periods in your self-created hectic life programme. Create stress-free breathing spaces during the course of the day, e.g. for doing isometric, relaxation or deep-breathing exercises. Try exercises that force you to slow down. *See* Appendix C for some office-based exercises.

Help yourself

Looking at the list you first made, begin to identify some things that you *enjoy* doing that you also find stressful. The key is to manage your time so that you can fit all these things in.

Make a list of all the things that you do in a typical day. Specify the time, the activity, whether you enjoy it or not, and whether you get any outside support for the activity, e.g. sharing driving or housework. Also list whether it is a physically or intellectually demanding activity, and if it takes place indoors or out.

Activity	Enjoy?	Support?	Category	Indoors	Outside

Spend some time analysing your day.

- Is there any activity you could usefully omit?
- Are there any tasks you could delegate or share?
- Try and balance your day so that you incorporate both physical and mental tasks: make sure that at least part of the day is spent in the open air.
- If there is an activity that you find creates more unnecessary physical tension in you, try to identify the cause and remedy it.
- Pay attention to the balance between the physical and mental demands on your life.

List what you like doing, and then do more of it. Then look at your list again and identify by letter those that:

- cost money – M
- that are free – F
- you do with other people – P
- you do alone – A.

Do at least one thing a week that does not cost money, e.g. reading a book, making a favourite meal. Now work out how to solve the irritants on our examples list. This could now read:

1   Time wasters – be assertive: ask them to leave.
2   Commuting – What don't I like? Rush? Nothing to do on the train – take a book/buy a personal stereo.
3   The telephone – screen (answer phone) and/or shield unwanted calls (secretary).
4   The partner – be assertive: accept/deflect criticism.
5   Overrunning meetings – be assertive, ask to hold a meeting to discuss meeting management, rotate the chair.
6   Constant interruptions – see time wasters above, or ask secretary to shield.
7   Research career alternatives.

Other stress busters:

- Cultivate a *slower pace of living*. Do one thing at a time, and concentrate on it. Avoid collecting chores up, e.g. avoid making a phone call and surfing the net simultaneously.
- If relationships seem more trouble than there are worth, try and tackle the problem at source. Is it lack of time? Poor communication?
- Put aside time from all your other activities to give to yourself.
- Remember that your partner, friends and family can provide you with a great deal of energy, affection and emotional support. Bank yourself up with these and you should be able to fight any problem facing you.
- *Be open about your feelings*, especially anger or fear.
- *Learn to be assertive*: learn to ask for what you want, and how to say 'No'.
- If you *follow a religion* do not feel guilty about gaining strength from your beliefs.
- *Share your problems* with the people who are important to you, without over-burdening either yourself or them. A problem shared is a problem halved.
- Take up yoga – a useful anti-stress weapon, being both physically demanding and non-competitive.
- Deal immediately with any evidence of harassment or bullying at work.
- Programme yourself for change. Sign on for a meditation class; take up karate.
- Give yourself some *constructive self-talk* or positive affirmations ('I am good at my job/a good parent/have a good sense of humour'). Say these aloud, regularly.
- *Change some attitudes*. You may not be able to change other people's behaviour, but you can change your own reaction to it.
- *Learn to deflect* irritating behaviours, simply by choosing to ignore them.
- *Brainstorm* solutions to your stress problems.
- Use *ranking* to make your choices clearer when making decisions. Identify the problem: you want to change jobs but cannot make that first move. List, on one side of the page, the reasons for wanting to change. On the other side list those reasons why you can't change. Give each reason a numerical weighting, then total up the scores.

See Appendix D for some other ways to combat stress. These include:

- talking more about your feelings
- writing in a personal journal about the hardest emotions for you
- sharing a stress interview with a colleague
- identifying and extending your support network
- learning and applying some counselling skills
- challenging destructive self-talk (cognitive reframing).

Some of the statistics on stress are disturbing. One in ten people in the UK will spend some time in a hospital for the mentally ill at least once in their life.

Many successful people are threatening their physical and mental well being by approaching 'burn out', a phrase that describes an overdose of stress factors perfectly. Burn out, and the symptoms of stress, are reversible. The sooner you start being kinder to yourself, the better.

Finally, it may be worth considering these holy orders for a stress-free life.[8]

- Thou shalt not try to be all things to all people.
- Thou shalt not be perfect or even try.
- Thou shalt leave undone things that ought to be done.
- Thou shalt not spread thyself too thin.
- Thou shalt learn to say no.
- Thou shalt schedule time for thyself and thy supportive network.
- Thou shalt switch off and do nothing regularly.
- Thou shalt be boring, inelegant, untidy and unattractive at times.
- Thou shalt not feel guilty.
- Thou shalt not be thine own worst enemy.

References

1   Editorial (2000) Practice managers stressed and depressed. *Practice Manager*. **May**: 7.

2   Bhattacharya S (2001) GP burnout poses threat to implementation of NHS Plan. *Pulse*. July, p. 3.

3   Collins G (1985) *Spotlight on Stress*. Vision House, London.

4   Cooper C, Cooper R and Eaker L (1988) *Living with Stress*. Penguin, Harmondsworth.

5   Dickson A (1982) *A Woman in Your Own Right*. Quartet Books, London.

6   Friedman M and Rosenman R (1985) Your Stress Profile: so you're a Type A? Company/Reed Employment Stress file. *Company Magazine*, London.

7   Garratt P and Kent A (1985) 11 Point Plan to Beat Stress. Company/Reed Employment Stress file. *Company Magazine*, London.

8   Edmondson C (2001) *Ministers Love Thyself: a self help guide*. Referenced by Lister S (2001) Holy Orders for a Stress Free Life. *The Times*. 26 January.

9   Powell J (1978) *The Secret of Staying in Love*. Argus Communications, London.

Further reading

Freudenberger J (1983) *Burn Out: how to beat the high cost of success*. Bantam Books, New York.

Appendix A

Identifying the level of personal stress

Consider each of the following events and if they currently affect you, list the LCU (Life Change Unit) points and add them together.

1	Death of spouse	100
2	Divorce	73
3	Marital separation	65
4	Jail term	63
5	Death of close family member	63
6	Personal injury or illness	53
7	Marriage	50
8	Fired at work	47
9	Marital reconciliation	45
10	Retirement	45
11	Change in health of family member	44
12	Pregnancy	40
13	Sex difficulties	39
14	Gain of new family member	39
15	Business readjustment	39
16	Change in financial state	38
17	Death of close friend	37
18	Change to different line of work	36
19	Change in number of arguments with spouse	35
20	Mortgage over £10 000	31
21	Foreclosure of mortgage or loan	30
22	Change in responsibilities at work	29
23	Son or daughter leaving home	29
24	Trouble with in-laws	29
25	Outstanding personal achievement	28
26	Wife begins or stops work	26
27	Begin or end school	26
28	Change in living conditions	25
29	Revision of personal habits	24
30	Trouble with boss	23
31	Change in work hours or conditions	20
32	Change in residence	20
33	Change in schools	20
34	Change in recreation	19

35	Change in church activities	19
36	Change in social activities	18
37	Mortgage or loan less than £10 000	17
38	Change in sleeping habits	16
39	Change in number of family get-togethers	15
40	Change in eating habits	15
41	Vacation	13
42	Christmas	12
43	Minor violation of the law	11

According to Professor Holmes' research if your score is less than 150, there is only one chance in three that you will have a serious change in your health during the next two years. If you score between 150 and 300 your chances rise to about 50/50. If your score is over 300 points – be careful, there is an 80% chance for a major health change in the next two years. (Extract from *Spotlight on Stress* by Gary R Collins, PhD (Vision House).)

Appendix B

How vulnerable are you to stress?

This test was developed by psychologists Lyn Miller and Alma Dell Smith from Boston University Medical Centre in 1984.

Score each item: 1 = almost always, 5 = never.

	SCORE
I eat at least one balanced meal a day.	1
I get seven to eight hours' sleep at least four nights a week.	1
I give and receive affection regularly.	1
I have at least one relative within 50 miles on whom I can rely.	1
I exercise to the point of perspiration at least twice a week.	5
I smoke less than 10 cigarettes a day.	1
I take fewer than five alcoholic drinks a week.	1
I am appropriate weight for my height.	5
I have an income adequate to meet basic expenses.	1
I get strength from my religious beliefs.	4
I regularly attend club or social activities.	3
I have a network of friends to confide in about personal matters.	1
I am in good health.	1
I am able to speak openly about my feelings when angry or worried.	1
I have regular conversations with the people I live with about domestic problems, e.g. chores, money, and daily living worries.	1
I do something for fun at least once a week.	1
I am able to organise my time effectively.	2
I drink fewer than three cups of coffee (tea, cola) a day.	1
I take quiet time for myself during the day.	1
TOTAL	33

To get your score add up your figures and subtract 20. Any number over 30 indicates a vulnerability to stress. You are seriously vulnerable if you score in between 50 and 75, and extremely vulnerable if it is over 75. Time to review your life style?

Appendix C

When you're under stress, relaxation often requires a conscious effort. Develop reflective periods in your self-created hectic life programme. Try exercises that force you to slow down:

Here are some office-based exercises:

- massage the fingers of each hand in turn
- rub your scalp with your fingertips, concentrating on the hairline
- place the fingers of both hands on either side of the back of your neck, press and move them slowly outwards from the centre, breathing deeply
- eye rolling: start by 'looking' very slowly round your field of vision in a clockwise direction, repeat anti-clockwise
- close your eyes; stroke them with your fingertips ten times
- stand with legs slightly apart, and shake out tension from hands and lower arms
- take a *deep breath and exhale slowly*; imagine you are releasing the pent-up energy with every breath out
- roll your head slowly, or hunch your shoulders up towards your neck and then release
- alternately tense then release muscle groups
- *massage*: some therapists provide a home or work visiting service; this can be an ideal solution for busy workers
- try to get seven to eight hours sleep at least four nights a week; it is possible to 'catch up' on sleep: have an early night, following a long bath, let the answer phone take your calls
- *meditation*: meditation is a way of calming or stilling your mind even further than relaxation does, it is a deeper and fuller form of relaxation; it is, therefore, more fulfilling and better for you; choose a form of meditation that suits you, not all methods suit everyone
- *guided fantasy*: imagine yourself in a beautiful place; again, choose a place that is right for you: it may be a hot sunny beach, it may be a cool moonlit night, it may be a grassy riverbank; take yourself on a journey through your imagination and see what happens
- *Self-massage*: give yourself a quick 'lift' by massaging trouble spots at any time, without the use of lotions; imagine as you massage that you are dispelling all the tension and energy out from your body into the air around you. Massage should not be a hurried thing.

Take time out before and after for rest and relaxation or meditation; otherwise you are negating the effect.

Appendix D

Involve other people

Talk about your feelings with your partner or close friends.[9] Write in and exchange personal journals in which you identify and describe your feelings and attitudes in more detail. You and your partner/friend should spend five or ten minutes a day writing down some of the emotions and feelings generated by difficult situations. Then spend another ten minutes exchanging your thoughts. It is often easier to expose yourself on paper; and the paper does not interrupt, look critical or bored.

It may be easier to decide on a series of topics to write about, e.g:

*   What was the nicest thing that has ever happened to you?
*   What was the most devastating?

Add other topics: How do you feel about growing old? What is the hardest emotion to share? Do the words 'commitment' and 'responsibility' scare you? Who does/has provided you with the most emotional support in your lifetime? What is the hardest emotion for you to share?

Choose an adjective to discuss what these words mean to you:

*   Friendship
*   Hurt
*   Inadequate
*   Domineering
*   Confident
*   Uncertain
*   Unappreciated
*   Sympathy
*   Proud.

Try and recall the incidents when these emotions have surfaced.

Identify your support network

A problem for many of us is that we often expect most, or all, of our support to come from our immediate family. Extend your support network so that there is more choice in a crisis; and less emotional dependence on one or two people. List different types of support:

*   someone I can depend on to give me constructive criticism
*   someone I feel really close to
*   someone who introduces me to new people and ideas

- someone I enjoy chatting to
- someone who makes me feel competent and valued
- someone who is always a valuable source of information
- someone who will challenge me to sit up and take a good look at myself
- someone I can depend upon in a crisis
- someone I can share bad news with
- someone I can share good news and good feelings with.

You may find that your support network will be different for home and work problems. Once you have compiled the list you will be able to use friends, colleagues or acquaintances for more than just a sounding board for your circuitous problems. Very rarely does one person provide all the different levels of support equally well.

Learn some counselling skills[9]

The stress interview

Ask a friend to 'interview' you by asking leading questions about a stressful experience. They can write down the responses and may prompt you by saying such things as:

'Tell me more about that.'
'How did you feel then?'
'Is there anything else you want to say about the incident?'

He or she is not permitted to comment, give advice or criticise, but just give attention and support. They may not need to say or do anything but give you time to talk; you will know the answers yourself but just need time to sort them out. The interviewer asks the following questions:

Q1 Think about something that happened to you that was a very stressful experience for you. Tell me about it.
Q2 Was this something you knew was going to happen or was it a surprise to you?
Q3 What did you feel when this happened and what did you do?
Q4 Can you remember doing anything that made you feel any better or less anxious? Describe what you did.
Q5 Did you turn to anyone else for help?
Q6 If you had that to face again would you do anything different now? Could you have done anything to prevent this happening or that would have made it less stressful for you?
Q7 Did you learn anything about yourself as a result of the experience?

Co-counselling

Take it in turn to *listen* to each other *without* commenting or giving advice. Take about ten minutes each: do not allow the session to degenerate into a mutual chat.

Challenge destructive self-talk (cognitive reframing)[5]

Remember the last time you felt bad about something: angry, jealous, resentful, etc. What were you telling yourself? We often have a series of very destructive beliefs, many of which have been handed down from our parents. They are destructive because they mean we set impossibly high targets for ourselves that are impossible to attain. Think about some of these beliefs, and then challenge them logically. Destructive talk is judgemental and may well include unfair condemnation of yourself.

Destructive: I must be liked or loved by everyone.
Constructive: I don't like everyone, so why should everyone like me?
                       I love and am loved by a chosen few.

Destructive: Disagreement and conflict are a disaster and must be avoided at all costs.
Constructive: I can learn from conflicts, it is possible to disagree and still remain friends.

Destructive: I must be perfect.
Constructive: Perfection is impossible to attain. The world is not perfect, nor can we be.

Destructive: Other people exist to make us happy and we cannot be happy unless they do.
Constructive: Happiness comes from within.

CHAPTER 11

Goal setting and change management

In this chapter we look at how to use your advanced communication and assertiveness skills to plan, set goals and manage change.

Anyone working in health has had to learn to adapt, and learn fast. Careers are reshaped and additional responsibilities are accepted, the work changes in both style and content. Good management is proactive rather than reactive; so it is anticipated that those organisations that will succeed will be those who have actively prepared for change – change is unsuccessful when it has been improvised and forced rather than planned. There is no magic formula for change management, but there are some clear themes which include:[1]

- a clear sense of direction
- good communication
- strong feedback from service users
- robust performance management systems.

One of the early lessons of the 'best value' regime in local government has been that many public sectors lack even the most basic data necessary to inform change management.

To develop, people and organisations need to:

- be experimental and flexible
- keep informed of, measure and monitor trends and developments within their profession
- assess changes and developments in attitudes and behaviour of competitors, patients and society.

Managing change

Change is an inescapable part of our working lives, and yet most people resist change.

* What is change?
* Why do we need to change?
* How can you overcome resistance to change?
* How can you manage change and set goals?

Change is a constant in the workplace and world. To survive and grow we must adjust to change. Change is also messy and risky. Just when you think you've arrived you find you have hardly begun. Change is the key to progress but we resist it. Why? Because people react differently to change and change can be unsettling.

If we assume no change, or try to escape it, our choices will be harsher. We need to adapt to a turbulent world. The less sensitive and less proactive are lost.

We have already seen some changes operating in our careers. There is a movement from boss–subordinate relationships towards procedures, which encourage staff to work in flexible groups of equals. Work is no longer permanent and long term, and reward is more closely allied to achievement.

Change has to be managed, and as with any management process it needs to be understood before it can be managed. We need to understand:

* how to plan for change
* how to implement change
* how to evaluate change.

Within this, we need to identify:

* the future that we desire
* some of the forces driving change
* our own reactions to change
* the size and shape of the work to be done.

Step 1: understand the need to change

Everyone in primary care must prepare themselves personally and professionally for changes ahead. Change is fundamental to progress; it is necessary for survival. The NHS is facing some big challenges. With yet another reorganisation on our hands with the transition from PCGs to PCTs, health authorities to strategic health authorities, everyone is looking at enormous changes in their own careers, their working style and job brief. Practices have already been participating in major organisational change as they prepare to become small businesses operating within a consortium instead of in isolation. In management, change is traditionally seen as common, rapid and huge in its effects; the public sector is no longer exempt.

It is not only the manager and the perceptions of his or her role, which need to change. Good communication within the practice will be increasingly important:

- people will need to be kept informed and abreast of changes in policy and workload
- new ideas must be regularly discussed and information shared
- new techniques must be tried out where appropriate
- everyone should be encouraged to raise issues affecting their work
- everyone must indicate as soon as possible if accepted practice is inappropriate
- innovation and adaptability must become part of everyday life.

Step 2: understand the resistance

Change is always problematic because it presents dilemmas and conflict, the need to:

- experiment v need to be right
- manage the present v managing the change
- manage uncertainty v certainty
- balance necessary bureaucracy v innovation
- look at what to focus on: external changes or internal changes.

There are no simple answers. Balances need to be struck, without compromising principles.

We need to understand that resistance to change is often the expression of insecurity and fear: it exposes people to uncertainty and may alter work patterns for the worse. It is, therefore, more acceptable when the objectives and application are understood and do not offer a threat to security.

What individual resistance to change do we know about?

Reasons not to change

What are your own reasons not to change?

Habit   Inconvenience   Own (biased) view of situation

Loss of individualisation   Cost of change   Threat to own power base

Financial implications   Fear of the unknown   Security is bedded in the past

- I don't have the time.
- We tried it five years ago and it didn't work.
- Everyone will blame me if it doesn't work.
- It's not in the plan.

Medical representatives have a secret code that classifies doctors. How do you best communicate change to each type?

- *Hares*: progressive, adventurous, believe in professional development and best practice. In selling to the hare, emphasise medicine and the patient, and show best evidence.
- *Dinosaurs*: reactionary, dissatisfied, resistant to change, old-fashioned. Show deference and respect, give support and sympathy.
- *Sheep*: conservative, traditional, conscientious, caring, avoids risk. Show respect, emphasise that this behaviour is standard, normal practice.
- *Wolves*: entrepreneurs; active, energetic, ambitious. They delegate responsibility and love change. Emphasise the dynamic aspects of the change and the benefits to the doctor and practice.

How do you react to change? Do you feel confident and excited or uncertain and frightened?

Step 3: identify the need for change

- Stay alert to the need for change.
- Consider where you are now.
- Consider where you want to be.

Step 4: plan for change

Effective change needs careful planning. Any personal change will affect those close to you, and they may feel threatened by the new you!

- Identify who will be opposed and therefore will not assist.
- Identify who will not oppose but still not assist.
- Identify who will want it to happen, and make it happen.
- Recognise where there is agreement and conflict.
- Examine your training needs.

Chart who you need to involve, highlighting those who will support or challenge the change, by placing stakeholders as spokes around the hub of a wheel.[2]

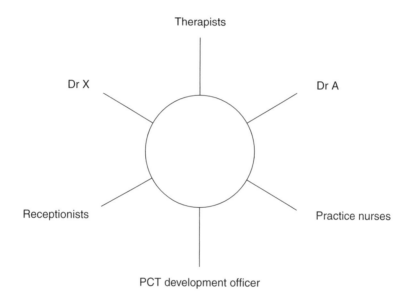

Step 5: monitor and evaluate

Check you have accomplished what you set out to do. Should the change be abandoned or adjusted? Talk to your team and find out.

You must keep routine work under control so there is time to innovate and implement the new ways of working. It has been said that managers must view change and innovation as opportunities to seize rather than as threats to fear. We will only learn to master change when we encourage, welcome and incorporate it into our personal and professional lifestyle. Those who do not fear change grow, learn, and continue to develop.

How to make change successful

Experiment. Be dynamic. Change is successful where:

- it has been preceded by other successful changes
- you have a clear set of cultural beliefs
- you take charge
- you have the energy, confidence and commitment to carry it through.

Successful change is organic, and dynamic and involves:

- innovation
- ice-breaking
- leadership
- vision
- strategy
- drivers.

Here are some pointers to assist you in managing the change process.

- Allow for a period of transition.
- Seek commitment and support.
- Seek out role models.
- Problem solve.
- Break things into steps: what needs to be done, when, by whom.
- Monitor your progress.
- Share your vision, your fundamental beliefs.
- Be honest with yourself.
- Listen to and understand the negatives.
- Acknowledge the history of organising things in a certain way, so any changes can be put on trial to see if they work.
- Use your supporters' energy, enthusiasm and lead.
- Preserve as many of the existing benefits as possible.
- Make people aware of the inevitable losses as well as the gains.
- Involve staff in identifying the need for change, and planning the new.
- Provide facts to avoid rumour and uncertainty.
- Provide reassurance.
- Communicate – keep an open door and an open mind.

Be aware of the effects of too much stress, and the effects of speedy change:

Shock → defensive withdrawal → acknowledgement → adaptation

You should allow for, and accommodate these feelings, and respond to them by encouraging those affected to seek support, attend self-awareness/development training programmes and counselling if necessary.

Change can be both painful and unacceptable to those who are not 'change masters'. Here are some pertinent observations on how **not** to manage change from a chief executive officer of a community health council involved in local consultations about local strategic issues.[3]

How not to manage change

- Assume everyone will understand and accept the need for change straight-away.
- Do not explain immediately, openly and clearly what you want to do and why.
- Allow time for rumours to circulate in order to increase anxiety and instability among the workforce and service users, and let these rumours reach the press before releasing your definitive plan.
- Be surprised and hurt when other groups attack or question your intentions: regard all resistance as an unfortunate obstacle to be overcome.
- If people express concerns which conflict with your own, console yourself with the thought that (a) they are troublemakers and not representative, (b) they cannot understand that what you want to do is the best thing and (c) there are Luddites in every age who are always going to dislike change however necessary or desirable it is.
- Do not base your plans on accurate information and predictions.
- Always let your timescale slip for release of plans and their implementation – this ensures lack of impetus.
- Do not allow time for effective consultation, ask people their opinions and then take no notice of them.
- Never answer letters or queries from outside interested parties. This makes people feel powerless and unheard.
- If you have to respond in some way, do so late so they can make no use of any information you may provide.
- If you have to deal directly with angry interested parties, appear to take their concerns seriously, then get on with the real business of managing change. Do not allow their concerns to influence you – this could cloud your vision and might give them delusions of power.
- Reserve all initiatives for yourself – this also increases your power while enhancing the powerlessness of others – keep them guessing!
- Be economical with the truth about the reasons for change. Do not, for example, tell people you are effectively making cuts because you do not have enough money. Tell them instead that what you are doing is best for them.
- Leave the future of the workforce vague. This destabilises people at a personal level and hopefully quite a lot of them will seek employment elsewhere leaving more space and less opposition for the change you desire.

Clearly, if these attitudes and practice are applied, service users and workers will be effectively alienated and resistance to change will increase.

Goal setting

We need goals as they provide a basis for objectives, planning and control. They also:

- help develop individual commitment
- reduce uncertainty in decision making
- help to focus direction.[4]

Goals tell us where we want to go, objectives tell us how to get there.

What is it that prevents us from achieving goals?

Achievement can only happen with good organisation and forward planning. There are three main problems with setting targets in general practice.

1　As the majority of GPs' work is reactive, the ethos and culture is to manage reactively. Hence, in general practice changes are rarely planned.
2　Most problems in resources and services are highly complex: with interrelated problems and opportunities, a fast moving and unpredictable environment, and multiple interest groups. Many people have an interest in the target solution and all will have different opinions, biases and interests.
3　Practice managers are often selected for good organisational skills at an operational level.

How to prevent failure

Plan the change

Chaos and disruption are common features when change is unplanned, and this creates additional stress individually and throughout the practice. In order to minimise and manage the risk of failure, practices can learn to address the major strategic issues and not simply concentrate on the operational management issues. Managers need to:

- map their environment
- understand the core purpose of their business
- paint a vision of their future.

Not all visions will be compatible. Whoever takes on the management role within a practice needs to assist the process of agreement within the partnership to define mutually acceptable aims. If personal and organisational goals are met and integrated, you will develop a stronger sense of identity and feel valued.

Team work

Failure occurs when goals have not been set and agreed by the entire team. Ideas must be discussed and agreed before implementation. Change is difficult to manage at the best of times, but unless everyone is part of this type of discussion, sabotage is common.

- Find out the level of commitment, and allocate the responsibilities fairly.
- Talk through your ideas with interested stakeholders first.
- Check viability of the plan with your sponsors first.

Manage conflict

We now know that conflict is a normal, and inevitable, reality of management and organisational behaviour. Remember that everyone has different needs, expectations, differences and attributes, then discuss where the conflict lies. Make the process mutual and participative, and try not to judge.

Here is a step-by-step approach detailing how you can achieve your aim.

Get organised

How organised are you? Complete the chart in Appendix A. Seek out the possible causes for poor organisation, and solve the problem.

- Lack of goals – write them down.
- Confusion in priorities – put first things first.
- Unrealistic time estimates – allow more time; allow for interruptions.
- Impatience with detail – take time to get it right.
- Manage by crisis – distinguish between urgent/important.
- Over commitment – delegate more.
- Knowledge explosion – read selectively.
- Over surveillance of subordinates – look to results, not detail.
- Refusal to delegate – accept that delegation is vital.
- Enjoyment of socialising – do it elsewhere; hold stand-up conferences.
- Indecision – make decisions with incomplete facts.
- Lack of confidence in the facts – improve your fact-finding procedures.
- Fear of the consequences of a mistake – use mistakes as your learning process.
- Fear of subordinates' inadequacy – train, allow mistakes; replace if necessary.

Set goals

You will never regret any positive move you make, however small. What you certainly will regret is not trying. It has been said that people who never make mistakes never make anything. Goals should be:

- specific, precise
- measurable (cost, quality, quantity, timeliness)
- achievable within the timescale
- realistic (provide a challenge, stretch the employee)
- jointly established not imposed
- broken down into objectives
- planned: indicate priorities (must do, could do), subject to a deadline
- continually updated
- checked for success.

If a particular task or goal is important enough, it is usually achieved, irrespective of all the obstacles and difficulties. The art of good management is identifying which goals are important, and achieving them using the minimum possible resources and without unnecessary stress. If you are getting stuck, use these ideas to assist you set goals.

BRAINSTORM

Brainstorm some solutions to long-standing problems

Then write down any that, in retrospect, you feel would work

Write down those that you would not consider

Are there any left over you are not sure about? Do not dismiss them.
Make a note of them here and come back to them at a later date

Write or draw the consequences of some of the solutions you are considering:

Develop positive thinking

List those areas where you can develop and improve, e.g. learn to listen more, sign up for assertiveness training.

1   *Achievements*. List all those things you are proud of. Be positive: 'at least I stuck that out for a year' is more optimistic than 'I always fail at any new training I try to do'.

2   *Core value system*. List five or more values that are important to you. Common examples include love, health, success, children and freedom. Order these from one to ten. Compare this list with your life now, or how you are planning your life. Are you living your life as you should? Are you planning your life with integrity?

   Know your own values. List your personal values. When we live in conflict with our own inner values, it can lead to unhappiness, frustration and blocks. Becoming aware of your values and prioritising them, helps you to reassess your goals.

   Start by making a list of ten values that you feel are important to you. Some common examples include: love, security, respect, money, achievement, health, success, ambition, freedom, integrity, compassion, independence, family, children, travel and trust. Next, try to put your own values in order, from 1 to 10. This can be difficult, and you may need to rework your list a few times before you feel it really reflects how you think and feel. Once you have done that, look at what the list is telling you. For example, if security, commitment and loyalty are high on your list, and you're working on short-term contracts, you are behaving in opposition to your values, and it will never make you happy. If freedom, independence and achievement are high on your list, you will need to be in a job that can give these qualities.

3   *Think of a solution to a problem.* The items can be as large or small as you
    wish – use them to form a checklist of things done/to do.

List all the things you would like to achieve over your lifetime

List those you could reasonably achieve within ten years

List those you will achieve this year

---

4   *Identify your current position.* Write down the numbers 1 to 10 in a
    straight line: 1 is very negative, 10 is very positive. Circle the number that
    describes how you currently feel about your situation. This gives a state-
    ment of where you are to start working.
5   *List these headings*: goals, personal strengths, immediate challenges/blocks/
    problems, development skills and achievements. Complete this using
    these guidelines:
    •   **Goals**: Goals are the foundation stones. Make these positive: some-
        thing you want to gain, not something you want to get rid of.
        Describe a goal, not a problem.
    •   **Personal strengths**: Concentrate on your strengths, not your weak-
        nesses. Don't downgrade your strengths. Believe you are worthy of
        what you want to achieve. Listing your strengths is a good way to
        focus on what you have to offer.
    •   **Immediate challenges/blocks/problems**: Focus on problems that
        directly affect you – don't list problems that blame or involve other
        people. You cannot think or make goals for other people, only for
        yourself, so don't write: 'to get partner X to work less hard, then they
        can pay more attention to my ideas'. Although your goal may well
        involve your partner, you cannot think or make goals for them, only
        for yourself. Consider the problem from another angle: Is there a way
        you can accommodate those long hours? Fill them with something
        absorbing and stimulating, so the absence bothers you less. Consider
        that you seem to find yourself attracted to people who treat you
        badly. Then you see the problem in a way that gives you control over
        solving it.

- **Development skills**: This is an area you can develop and improve. Listing these is a great way to focus on ways you can move forward. You are recognising that it takes two to communicate, and that you will take responsibility for the part you play. You might write 'learn to listen more', 'improve communication skills' or 'learn to be more independent'.
- **Achievements**: List achievements you are proud of, positively: instead of 'I found the strength to leave a bad job and look for a good one', try 'I am always willing to tackle problems and take risks'. Your achievements list is a great prompt to move you forward because it makes you ask yourself the right questions, and to keep you positive and solution-oriented.
  - What have I learnt from this?
  - How have I progressed?
  - What have I gained?
  - How would I do things differently next time?[5]

Finding the solution

Keep the *focus on your own place in the problem*. Ask yourself positive, self-focused and solution-focused questions – 'How can I ask questions in a way that X doesn't find threatening?'. But relationships often present complicated problems. If you find it difficult to see a way past the problem, try the doorway technique. *Brainstorm* every solution. Close your eyes and imagine each solution written on a doorway. Stand in front of one of the doors and walk through it. What's on the other side? If you don't like it, you can walk back through the door and try another one. Visualisation can be an unnerving but very powerful tool, which helps you to see just what you most fear from making a particular decision. Using visualisation lets you walk through the doors again and again, until it looks less threatening. Keep asking yourself the right questions. How can I make this work for me? How can I turn this situation around?

Audit your success

Having defined your goals and planned their implementation, the next step is to audit your success in meeting them. Goal analysis enables you to break down such instructions or goals into specific actions. These can then be used to measure how well the requirements are met, to audit qualitative criteria.

The first step is to *clarify your goal*. The question 'How do patients respond when they are made to feel welcome?' might produce a list such as the following:

- happy
- comfortable

- satisfied
- approving
- appreciated
- amiable.

Check each item for relevance and importance. For example, you might discard 'amiable' as being unimportant, and 'happy' as being irrelevant as an unhappy patient can still be made to feel welcome.

Having established how you would like your patients to feel in order for this goal to be met, next write down any action which would contribute to this. *Identify the behaviour.*

Having identified the behaviour that produces the required results, you may wish to *set a specific target* for that behaviour to be repeated, e.g. 'Receptionists to alert patients of the appointment delay time every hour'. Aim to measure quality as well as quantity.

At times you may find that your attempts to analyse a certain goal get bogged down. You may end up chasing a different goal or even giving up the analysis. This does not necessarily mean that you are doing anything wrong. You will find out which ones are unnecessary, inappropriate or elusive.

The above method of goal analysis enables you to measure, to a greater or lesser degree, your achievements in meeting goals which are difficult to quantify. Those that can be checked against a graph or spreadsheet are simpler but no less important; it is essential that regular reviews be conducted to monitor the state and progress of all the practice goals.

- What are you currently doing towards meeting your present goal?
- What do you plan to do next year?

Planning

Good planning is essential to a smooth-running, communicating organisation. The *process* of planning enables you to:

- see clearly where you are at present
- clarify some of the wider issues facing you or your organisation
- firm up any new proposals
- evaluate yourself and the organisation
- provide a statement of intent for interested stakeholders
- formulate goals
- identify the action needed to achieve these goals
- identify resources required in terms of skills, activity and finance
- anticipate ahead
- ensure the negotiation of the best possible funding.

How do we plan?

- Identify the problem.
- Collect the data to quantify the problem.
- Analyse the problem.
- Organise and coordinate a plan of action.
- Implement.
- Review.
- Monitor.

Good planning involves:

- objectivity
- realism
- flexibility
- logical thinking
- wide communication
- everyone's involvement
- delegation
- team work
- time.

Have you got this in your team?

Use a chart to plan

If you are moving premises, for example, try planning the stages using a chart, with the goals on the vertical axis, and the timescale on the horizontal:

Goals	Timescale by:			
	1 Aug	7 Aug	14 Aug	21 Aug
Contact solicitors	✔			
Alert and publicise to stakeholders				✔
Change publicity		✔		
Plan removal	✔			
Sell unwanted equipment				✔
Confirm change to computer company		✔		
Confirm removal date			✔	
Contact utilities				✔

Projects

When writing a project brief take the reader step-by-step through the process:

- a proposal
- detail of the project
- ways of evaluating the performance.

It is important to ensure consistency and focus through the project's life cycle. One way of doing this is to prioritise goals and objectives with specific indicators: must do, could do. You must do something if the risk to the organisation or project is high; but not if the impact is low. This example looks at the risk of not managing the risk of a burglary within a practice.

Risk	Probability	Impact
Of burglary if practice unsecured	High	High: insurance/disruption costs
PCT will not reimburse	High	Low: practice will pay
Threat to staff	Low	High
No real financial gain	High	High

Remember: *Prior planning prevents poor performance.*

Objectives and targets

Here is a selection of the aims one manager set for herself:

- improve communication with staff
- select different chair for meetings
- need to learn more about working strategically not operationally
- delegate more!
- need to improve financial management skills and develop appropriate management systems.

How does this fit into a plan? Once you have identified your priorities, and have costed them, then stage them, marking each target with an aim (what the plan is) and objective (how to map the outcome).

- Detail your targets for the year to come.
- Note how success will be measured once the object has been achieved.
- Note who is responsible for achieving it by when: using basic 'who', 'why', 'what', 'where', 'when' headings. Note the cost, if any, of your plan, and when you hope to achieve it by.
- Be specific and clear about your objectives.

Then consider how these aims should be prioritised, how success will be measured once the object has been achieved, and who is responsible for achieving it by when. With the date, cost and achieved date noted, you have a complete record of the process. *See* Appendix B if you tend to procrastinate.

Objectives, like goals, should be:

- measurable
- realistic and achievable
- time bound.

Note also any critical success factors, and build in a system for monitoring whether or not you have achieved your objectives. Use the following table as a template.

Objective/target	How will you measure success	Who is responsible	Date for action	Cost	Achieved by

References

1   Brindle D (2001) Clear Sighted. *Guardian Society.* 11 July, p. 12.

2   Turrill T (1986) *Change and Innovation in the NHS.* Management Series 10, The Institute of Health Service Management, 75 Portland Place, London WIN 4AN. Tel: 020 7637 2311.

3   Pattison S (1991) Masters of Change. *Health Service Journal.* 31 October, p. 23.

4   Kast F and Rosenzweig J (1985) *Organisation and Management: a systems and contingency approach* (4e). McGraw-Hill, London.

5   (2000) New You. *The Observer.* 9 January, pp. 36–9.

Further reading

Change Here! The Audit Commission Publications. Tel: 0800 502030 or www.audit-commission.gov.uk/changehere.

Carter R *et al.* (1984) *Systems, Management and Change – a graphic guide.* Paul Chapman Publishing/Open University, London.

Appendix A

Personal organisation

For the factors below circle a number that most represents your views of your organisation.

1 I am ruthless with paperwork. I only keep top priority paperwork for the time it is needed.	1 2 3 4 5	I have never thought about paperwork. I tend to keep all of it for too long.
2 I have now developed a desk organisation system based upon my top priority work.	1 2 3 4 5	My desk organisation system is haphazard; often it is non-existent.
3 Normally I can retrieve information quickly from my system.	1 2 3 4 5	I normally have to search a great deal for my information. Sometimes I lose essential pieces of information.
4 I use my desk for *working* on and I operate a *clear desk* policy.	1 2 3 4 5	I use my desk to *store* work on. I don't operate a *clear desk* policy.
5 When I am working on top priority work I make sure that I will not be interrupted unless it is a top priority interruption.	1 2 3 4 5	When I am working on top priority work I am often interrupted. I have difficulty in dealing with these interruptions.
6 I very rarely give *priority* to an interruption.	1 2 3 4 5	Normally interruptions do take *priority* over the work I am doing at the time.
7 In my work team we have established a 'code of practice' on interruptions.	1 2 3 4 5	We have no 'code of practice' for interruptions in my work team.
8 I always batch my telephone calls into top and low priority.	1 2 3 4 5	I have no priority system for telephone calls and I do them at any time during the day.
9 For top priority work I never rely on being rung back. I make appointments to ring back again until I have the information.	1 2 3 4 5	For top priority work I always ask the manager to ring me back if not available or if information is not available.
10 My opening line in a telephone call is my name, purpose and action.	1 2 3 4 5	My opening line in a telephone call is my name.
11 I often hold long telephone conversations on top priority work in preference to a meeting.	1 2 3 4 5	I very rarely hold long telephone conversations on top priority work. Meetings are preferable.
12 For much of my lower priority work my secretary or subordinate will handle it directly.	1 2 3 4 5	I have not briefed my secretary or subordinates on handling lower priority work.

Appendix B

How to avoid procrastination

Successful approaches for difficult tasks:

- Use the five-minute brainstorm: break the project down into smaller activities and write these down.
- Focus attention on the smaller individual activities: concentrate on the smaller, bit-sized pieces to avoid feeling overwhelmed.
- Block out an adequate length of time: don't start work just before lunch or meetings; it will only reinforce your negative feelings.
- Work when you are at your best: reserve quality time for important jobs and do the low payoff tasks after lunch and at other low times.
- Start each session with something easy: do anything to get going rather than nothing at all.
- Redefine the project: others may have ideas to simplify it. Remember: it is better to deliver a simple one on time than not deliver a complex one.

Successful approaches for long-term tasks:

- Determine a realistic time commitment per week: it is better to set and stick to an hour a week than set ten hours and do nothing. Even the largest project will respond to steady progress.
- Specify tasks in advance: end each session by specifying the next session's work. This enables your subconscious to work on it and also makes it easier to get started next time.
- Establish a regular time for working on long-term projects: it will help make it become a habit.
- Establish deadlines for intermediate progress points: set self-imposed deadlines for short-term activities which can be completed in a week or less.
- Switch to other aspects of the overall task: prevent boredom or frustration by working on different areas of the project.
- Avoid the activity trap: don't lose sight of the long-term goal.
- Limit the number of major projects: remember that routine activities will take up a large proportion of your time.
- Record your on-going progress each week: any form of diary, calendar or graph can be used to show that you are making progress.
- Improve efficiency by grouping similar tasks.
- Break up tasks into manageable chunks.
- Use titbits of time: always have something to read or work on with you.
- Reduce interruptions and time leaks: set aside chunks of quality time and use them profitably.
- Avoid perfectionism: it costs too much.

CHAPTER 12

Developing your management skills

This last chapter identifies:

- how you can apply assertiveness skills to develop yourself and your relationships at work
- some of the behaviours of good and bad managers
- some of the skills you may need to acquire if you are seeking promotion
- those skills you need to develop to gain more respect for your present abilities
- those skills required to manage your boss and colleagues more effectively.

If you know yourself better, you are more likely to be able to take control of your life, and live it actively rather than passively. As you take on more responsibility, a different kind of respect is demanded which has both financial and personal implications. Those unused to this new role may need to learn new personal skills to support their new sense of self. Learn to take charge!

Moving on and up

- Does your work provide you with opportunities for growth and learning?
- Will you get bored with what you're doing in the next five – or 15 years?
- Are the salaries at your job level sufficient for you to be able to provide for both your present and future financial needs by yourself?
- How much authority do you have to make decisions?
- Does your job adversely influence your home life?
- Do you feel that you are making a worthwhile contribution through your work?

Doing good work at the moment will get you recognised, but it may not be enough to get you promoted, because jobs at different levels call for very different qualities and skills. You may be intelligent, competent and skilled at what you do but ask yourself: What does my superior do that I don't?

Put aside your own prejudices. It is simplistic to think that managers waste time on the phone all day long talking to their friends, as the friends may be crucial connections whose ideas are vital to the job. Learn to network and build relationships:

* join professional organisations and take an active role in them
* use every phone conversation and every meeting as a chance to make contacts
* take the time to talk with people so that vital relationships can grow
* learn from these connections and pass information onto your boss
* introduce your boss to important connections.

Convince your employer that you have the higher-level capabilities they are looking for if you are seeking promotion, people don't take risks on unproven quality. You should:

* analyse the job for which you are aiming
* look at what the people at that level are doing
* locate the key qualities and skills required.

If you think you are not being promoted because your manager won't acknowledge how you have changed, you haven't changed in a way that is essential for success at the next level. If you feel you are seen in 'the same old way', consider the following points:

* how do you think your organisation views you at work?
* what kind of person do they promote?
* what are the qualities in these people? Enthusiasm? Confidence? Ability to motivate?
* do they see that you have the necessary qualities for promotion?
* make a list of your possible weaknesses and analyse them.
* do any of them present major handicaps at the next level?

Once you've determined what characteristic might be holding you back, decide if you value the quality, or if you want to change.

Never accept more responsibility without the corresponding job title. Many smaller organisations still exploit women through the limited opportunities they have to do challenging work – but the reward of flattery is not enough. Negotiate a pay rise. You are entitled to have the title to match what you are doing so that your responsibilities are clear to people both internally and externally. Your employer's negotiating strength is based on giving you the opportunity you want so badly, and your strength is behaving as if you are a gift to them: they want you to do the new work. It's not easy to replace someone who knows the ropes; it is time-consuming, costly and risky.

Promotion within the same organisation: the new manager

Once you have been newly promoted, your working methods will need to change, as taking on a new management position will result in the development of new loyalties. Previously the organisation may have been considered in terms of what it could do for you. You now need to address what is good for the organisation, for your employees, and yourself.

Your job subtly changes:

- the things you used to do are taken out of your hands
- the working relationships change
- you will be learning the new job while you are training others into your old job
- you redefine your creativity within a wider framework
- you can still do the work better than most people, only now you can tell others how to do it better as well.

The way you first approach your new employees will make the difference between whether or not you will be effective as a leader. There are several diplomatic basics that a manager must bear in mind if he or she wants to be successful at it, and they are essential to doing the job.

Tips for the new boss

- Firstly, assert the fact that you are the boss.
- Present yourself as a new person welcoming the people who are already there.
- Set a cordial formal friendliness at the start but don't isolate yourself: you need to develop relationships and insights into the way people think.
- First identify with and relate to your peers: it may be nice to have the post room people on your side, but they still have to deliver your mail whether you expend a lot of energy on them or not.
- Remember you represent your title as well as yourself, and do not be afraid to use the clout of that title to demand a certain respect.

If managing friends:

- acknowledge and discuss the difficulties with them honestly
- try to get a pledge of commitment to work towards a positive goal
- consider how others may view the friendship
- be alert to taking out frustrations on friends, you both know each other's weaknesses.

If managing older/more experienced colleagues:

- tap into their experience and knowledge of the organisation
- try for a pledge of non-competition
- their age and length of service equals commitment, get them involved
- seek out their assistance when training/mentoring new staff.

Wanting to be liked

Being liked is not a key to functioning well in the job. It's much more important to engender a sense of respect for yourself as a professional. If you are seen as too friendly, staff will take up too much of your time. Provide a place where your people can work and express their talents to the full, and you will be considered a good boss.

Acceptance and rejection

The need for acceptance is a powerful factor in the human psychology, as is the fear of rejection. When you compliment someone who works for you, you are using a powerful tool in building loyalties and improving motivation. When you comment negatively on an employee's work, you are playing on a fear of rejection. Under such psychological pressure people are not able to perform as well as their best, and may seek to undermine your position. Be assertive:

- do not use the threat of termination to whip staff into line – people respond better to positive tactics
- create a situation where people want to come to work: you will have fewer problems with resentments, fewer demands for pay increases and fewer complaints about conditions.

Competence

- Instil a sense of being in charge by handling the problems that come your way
- If your staff trust you they will feel more comfortable and more motivated to do their best.

If you have quirks, make them predictable personality traits and not sudden demonstrations of irrational behaviour. Your staff must believe that you are capable of doing your job, since how you do it affects how they do theirs. Don't create scenes: especially over the working habits of people who are working well overall. It outrages them, spoils their focus, wrecks their enthusiasm, and destroys your credibility.

Problem solving

You must develop a technique to arrive at solutions.[1]

- If the problem involves a direct work situation, make a decision based on your experience.
- Use other people's experience to assist: discuss problems and their solutions collectively.
- Your forte as a boss is to be able to recognise the solution and 'decide' on it.
- You don't have to have the answers – just the ability to find them.

If a problem develops, it now becomes your job to find out whether the system is at fault or the people:

- ask and listen: those doing the job are best qualified to tell you where the inefficiencies are
- never ignore problems that don't seem to be your province
- if there are unclear and unspoken resentments about co-workers, and efficiency is affected, take appropriate steps.

What constitutes a good boss?

Good managers:

- *Delegate responsibly*. Work completed as scheduled demonstrates whether staff are working efficiently, but never make unreasonable demands around a deadline. Make it clear that you understand that circumstances, not just incompetence or stupidity, cause delays: people who work under conditions free from blame make fewer mistakes.
- *Point out mistakes*, and allow for an explanation. Accept certain mistakes as inevitable; look for a solution together.
- Maintain a sense of the *outside world*. If your senior staff are producing and achieving well, don't worry so much about formalities such as nine-to-five punctuality. They are working for you and for themselves, too. Accept that some staff are using their job as a stepping-stone to another job – perhaps yours – and that your own position is ultimately a temporary one.
- *Financial support*. Part of a manager's job is determining when an employee deserves a rise and handling the situation when this cannot be granted. As a manager, you sit between organisational policy and employees' needs. You cannot be a revolutionary and ruin your reputation with management, and you cannot alienate your staff by taking a hard line: present a fair and urgent appeal when there is a real need to get more money for

staff. Always keep people informed of your efforts, and if you can't ask for a rise at a particular time, be straightforward about it, providing honest suggestions if necessary.

- *Meetings* are the best way to gather ideas from the people most able to advise: make sure your staff see their value. A frequent exchange of ideas will help staff view one another's talents and maintain your position as the final authority. Emphasise the importance of meetings by the times you schedule them. Perhaps 10 am on Mondays to kick off the week. And expect people to be punctual.
- *Firing*. If you have to make this decision, do not allow guilt to invade the issue. It only places you in a vulnerable position and you may make concessions you'll regret. Actions such as firing, reprimanding or refusing rises do create emotional pressure and should be approached with the correct intent – that of maintaining the function and efficiency of your department. They should not be emotional decisions:
    - accept that firing people is part of being a boss
    - do not moralise or try to justify your actions
    - keep accurate documentation of the incidents that led you to your decision
    - don't give your ground if challenged
    - remember you have the right to demand competence from your staff.

Bad managers damage their staff's careers and invalidate their staff. There is no room in any organisation for managers who:

- *'Put down'*. Make subtle derogatory remarks that undercut self-confidence instead of helping the person gain an awareness of their talents. Talented people will be more willing to work for those who appreciate them: you will get better results and more recognition.
- *Threaten or bully*. Managers who do this reveal their own insecurities. People are not so scared that they can't see through such a ploy. Such behaviour is unacceptable.
- *Are inflexible*. Staff should be a unit of various ideas, plans, dreams and talents. A manager has the responsibility not only for making final decisions, but also for utilising the talents that they are being paid for. Find the merits in ideas and requests, and when you must refuse something do it with encouragement to continue generating new ideas.
- *Are timid*. Either they don't trust their own judgement or are afraid of being disliked. There is no place in business for a manager who cannot say no:
    - saying no does not stifle talents and creativity
    - if you do not take charge staff may gain so much ascendancy that they start to dictate what should be your prerogatives.

Points to remember

- Do not avoid difficult situations or accept mediocrity.
- Face your insecurities, and learn how to cope with authority.
- Listen, ask questions, take advice and then ACT.
- Allow yourself to make mistakes – assurance will come with experience.
- Remember that there is no such thing as the perfect boss.
- Bring yourself into the best focus possible.
- Remember that good intentions are as important as any other quality.
- You have the responsibility to use all your capabilities.

Plan your own career change

It is said that in life there are four types of people:

- people who watch things happen
- people to whom things happen
- people who don't know what is happening
- people who make things happen.

Are you concerned for your future? Do you feel your work is limiting you? Try these exercises that were developed by McGill and Beaty.[2] Give yourself some time to reflect when answering the following questions.

- WHO: mentally scan all the people who may be relevant to you, and what you may need to do to develop this network.
- WHAT are the key areas you can tackle quickly to provide early success.
- WHERE: reflect on your work and living environment.
- WHEN: timing is crucial. You need to be in the right place at the right time – when to act or not is a highly developed skill.
- HOW: Think about new, creative and innovative actions. Trust your intuition. The behaviour that caused the problem is unlikely to solve it.

Answer the following questions, asking yourself *why*.

Personal

- Do you pay sufficient attention to your personal needs?
- What support is available and do you use it well?
- What work pressures do you inflict upon yourself and family?
- How does your work enhance or detract from the quality of your life?
- Who controls how you use your time?

Professional

- Do you prefer to lead or be led?
- Do you prefer stability or initiating change?
- Do you know, or want to know how others perceive you? How can you find out?

Organisation

- What recent changes are affecting you most and how?
- In which areas of work do you feel most comfortable and uncomfortable?
- Why are you working in health services and what would make you want to leave?
- What opportunities does health offer you as a career? What are the expectations and constraints?
- How has your job changed over the past year?
- What did you achieve?
- What would you like to do more of?
- What does your past performance tell you about your strengths, weaknesses, and needs for training and development?
- What type of work would you ideally like to do?
- What are the key conditions you require to provide you with job satisfaction?

From answering these questions, what changes do you need to make? To impress potential employers you need to be able to demonstrate certain key skills which:

- will enhance your personal effectiveness
- can be learned and demonstrated
- will improve your employability
- will help enable you to move between jobs, maybe even between the public and private sectors.

It will be increasingly important for healthcare workers to demonstrate that they can take on any developmental and strategic work needed in their organisation. Through your present job you can demonstrate your ability to think analytically, show how you manage your time and prioritise your work. Employers especially value the following skills:

- communication and numeracy
- use of information technology
- continually improving one's own learning and performance.

Others cite ability to work with others and problem solving. These are the skills most in demand. Mark off those you already have, or can attain:

- team working
- interpersonal skills
- motivation
- enthusiasm
- flexibility
- customer awareness
- business awareness
- problem solving
- planning and organisation.

Take the time now to reflect on the skills you now have – in paid work and in any other area of your life. Can you demonstrate how, in your present job, you:

- cooperate with your fellow workers (team working)
- seek and build relationships with colleagues (networking)
- listen to and consider a range of opinions, explain alternatives and make recommendations (flexibility)
- handle complaints, take responsibility for interviewing and staff appraisals, chair meetings (interpersonal communication skills)
- manage finances (numeracy)
- use IT
- develop customer awareness (promotion of a patient participation group, or set up a proactive complaints procedure).

Use your CV as a medium for demonstrating these skills – mention sought after key words frequently: 'I am familiar with *planning services* and *organising* staff/GP workloads/appointment systems; I trust my awareness in *developing* primary care as a *business* will stand me in good stead ...'.

If you are an organiser with an eye on the future, someone who sees the big picture rather than detail, use language which indicates completion of a goal: active verbs (ending in *-ing*: organis*ing*, forward plann*ing*, problem solv*ing*). This demonstrates positivism, motivation and enthusiasm. It demonstrates the ability to plan ahead, problem solve and think strategically.

Passive verbs demonstrate your steadfastness and staying power. These verb endings indicate solidity and reliability on your CV and at an interview: 'I plan services, organise the appointment systems, solve problems as they present'. This indicates you feel more comfortable dealing with present crises rather than anticipating, looking to the future and strategising.

Most employers in the (still bureaucratic) public sector are still looking for completer-finishers – creativity and imagination are not commonly requested attributes. Entrepreneurs and opportunists are not generally sought after, but are needed to complement teams. GPs may need to seek a complement to their individualism. General practice tends to attract clinicians who prefer to work alone, or entrepreneurs – it may be advisable for their managers to balance these traits.

- Use language that accurately reflects your personal communication style so that your future employer can see if your face fits.
- Draw attention to other key personal qualities such as honesty, reliability and sensitivity.

Building a relationship with your manager

This relationship is critical because of the power your employer holds over you. You therefore need to both manage yourself and develop the relationship you have with your manager. If you want to succeed you need to manage your superiors and yourself.

Your boss may cause you problems and sometimes the greatest anxiety, but a boss can also be a mentor, giving you a wider view of the world. It is important to understand their world, values and problems. Your boss reports to someone just as you do, even chairs and chief executive officers report to the board of directors and ultimately to the shareholders and the public.

People succeed when they are motivated to work hard at something that singled them out. Without ambition there is little progress. However, more people have failed at work through not being able to fit in or establish good relationships on the job than for any other reason. Relationships, and good communication, are of the essence.

Tips for managing your boss

- Find out who your boss reports to. It will help to know what pressures and demands are put on your boss.
- Understand the responsibilities your boss has.
- Understand what your boss is dependent on you for – if you can help your boss to function well, you may make a powerful ally.
- See the relationship for what it is without the emotional overtones, then your ego will not be destroyed every time you are asked to do something you may not want to do.
- Deal with your boss with the same care and objectivity that you deal with associates and subordinates. Be a friend within the bounds of the relationship.
- Maintain communication: inform them of any problems, so that they are not surprised or unprepared for any consequences.
- Do not waste time relating trivial or non-essential matters to them.

Quantify your productivity

Learn to assess yourself and so increase your efficiency and effectiveness. Look at the cost of your work: the quantity, the quality and the time it takes to produce a certain amount of work. Quantify your value to the organisation using measurable factors:

- number of enquiries or presentations
- number of complaints
- the amount of income or profit generated through your activities.

Take outside work to develop yourself but first check:

- organisational policy on any restrictions to doing other work
- there is no conflict of interests
- if you need authority for a special dispensation.

You need to:

- be loyal – it is important to your integrity and to the trust placed in you
- set standards for yourself and better them
- plan
- prioritise.

Meetings

Have frequent meetings with your boss. It is not enough to have performance reviews once a year. A request for more frequent meetings is legitimate and shows your concern beyond the immediate task to be done; it demonstrates an attempt to understand the thinking and planning of upper management. Use the meeting to:

- check you are meeting objectives
- understand required standards of performance
- gain useful information about the needs of the organisation
- update your boss with information
- gain feedback so you can improve your performance
- confront difficult situations and solve problems together.

You have to decide when it's possible, practical and politic to use your superior to help solve a work problem and when to turn elsewhere. Then you won't be victimised by the real, or imagined, failings of your manager.

Under which circumstances do you feel failed by your manager and why?

My manager is always unavailable

They used to listen, communicate and be accessible, but now, whenever you try to see your manager, they are on the phone or shuffling papers; you feel overlooked and ignored. Consider that you may have disappointed or dissatisfied them and they have unassertively begun withdrawing their attention. They are not being assertive so you have to take the lead:

- ask: identify the problem
- are you creating extra work for your manager in some way?
- are you asking too many questions but not providing the recommendations, opinion or judgement required?
- make your own choices: 'Here's what I think we should do' instead of 'What should I do?'

Offer solutions to problems that have arisen while you are doing the assigned work, thus exercising your own initiative. It may strengthen your relationship with your boss and give you an edge when being considered for promotion. Finally, never ask your boss for information you can get from others. By keeping informed through other channels, you'll protect your image of being bright and on top of things. Use their time as efficiently and productively as your own.

My manager doesn't give me any direction

Your chief value lies in the extent of your ability to direct yourself. If you want to advance your career, you have to be able to take the initiative. Take this as an opportunity. You only need approval for your selected course of action.

I'm afraid to admit to mistakes

Errors are inevitable but women especially have a problem believing this, and hesitate to jump in without preparation, afraid of making a mistake. Men, however, have more confidence to go through a time of error-making to acquire their expertise. From an early age, women's efforts are focused on avoiding the errors that bring criticism.

- Acquire as much experience as you can.
- If you make an error, devise strategies to cover yourself.
- Learning from your errors is an important way of acquiring wisdom.

- Act quickly, do not procrastinate. Mistakes are better tolerated when people see that you understand your error and that you've taken steps to correct it.
- If you've made the mistake of not dealing with a problem immediately, act as if the delay had never occurred.

The job isn't what I thought it would be

Take care during the early days of your job, as job descriptions are often determined not in discussion during the interview, but in practice during the early days in the job.

- If you are asked to do anything that you do not consider your remit – say so. Strong managers can bully their staff into something unacceptable.
- Establish your job description then reject the new work.
- Demonstrate you are able to compromise and use your judgement, and that you will not be manipulated.

I don't look as if I'm on top of the job

When you move into a new job, it's important for you to be seen as strong and confident. Appear in command.

- Hand out short-term projects to each of your staff, so that you will quickly be able to judge their individual skills, and degree of competence and cooperativeness.
- Let everyone know that you are now in the judgement seat; that his or her previous reputations do not count for very much.
- Be quick to praise and criticise. Don't exhibit too much patience with those who don't deliver. When you move in strongly, you are acting to minimise the possibilities of future trouble.
- If people see you as a powerful force, they'll think twice about engaging in office combat with you and, instead, will seek out ways and means to ally themselves to you.

I can't get anything done

One of the biggest single stumbling blocks to getting things done in any new job can be the inability to make the right contacts. Your first concern should be people: who will back your ideas or resist them, who is happy to see you come in, and who resents you?

- Size up the different alliances before you get too friendly, and especially before you give them work.

- To win cooperation, court your colleagues assiduously, make lunch dates with them, throw them ideas they can use in their own work, offer insights and ask for their advice.

Building relationships with your colleagues

This relationship depends on the task to be performed. You and your colleagues:

- can be mutually interdependent, which means that neither could do the job alone
- may both work on the same projects simultaneously so a continuous dialogue is needed
- may be serially interdependent: one of you must finish a piece of the task before the other one can take it up
- may work side by side with the same overall production objective.

Mutual interdependence requires:

- good problem-solving ability
- a capacity to tolerate each other's working styles be they quick, slow, meticulous or creative
- you both to keep checking your tolerances and expectations of each other
- collaboration
- a sense of healthy, managed, competition.

Be assertive and check how well you are interacting at intervals: 'How do you think we are working together? I am satisfied with X, but feel we could improve on Y. How do you feel?' This strengthens equality, professional intimacy, mutual understanding, and communication of task-related thoughts and feelings.

Socialisation meets important needs; for many people it is a primary reason for enjoying work. Maximise your effectiveness and satisfaction by socialising 'up' as often as you can, socialise frequently 'horizontally' and once in a while socialise 'down', as well.

The main issue in *serial interdependence* is expectations:

- be sure that you and your colleague agree on the quality specifications and your deadlines
- voice any concerns about the quality or timing of a colleague's work early: tell the other person what you appreciate about their work, reinstate your expectations, and negotiate outcomes together.

Building relationships with subordinates

The dynamics of boss–subordinate relationships

A boss is in a position of power, and as such may be viewed as someone who clearly holds the power, and:

- whose needs are largely met by their subordinates
- who feels good, free and satisfied in the relationship
- who experiences no need to share feelings, opinions and judgements
- who implicitly keeps others doing all the difficult, 'feelings' work.

In this instance the subordinate may be less powerful and:

- spend a lot of energy assisting and supporting their boss
- take care of their perceived needs
- may lose track of their own needs
- can become resentful, frustrated and angry
- seek out support from peers or the same culture, race and sex
- withhold feelings and thoughts because of a perceived high risk.

A good boss should be aware of this power imbalance and work to know their subordinates well:

- their strengths and weaknesses
- how they work under pressure and collaborate as team members
- how they deal with ambiguity or unpredictability
- are they meticulous prodders? Sloppy but creative? Responsible, loyal, autonomous, ambitious?

If you don't know your staff you can't utilise their strengths and help develop their potential. Get to know people: spend time with them, work and talk with them, observe and reflect. There are two critical components in the relationship with subordinates. First, a manager needs to communicate clearly with them; second, they must know how and when to delegate responsibility to them. Keep checking with the person on what they are hearing, on how they are feeling about the content of the communication. We know that in communication the content is *what* is being said; the process is *how* it is being said. *See* the author's book: *Communication and the Manager's Job* (Radcliffe Medical Press, 2002) for more details.

Developing your management skills

Network

The grapevine reflects the opinions, hopes and anxieties of employees, and those who hope to know what is going on must learn to plug into it.

* Get out of your office, circulate and listen.
* Identify the opinion leaders and gossips.
* Become trusted. To get information, you must give information. And it must be sound.
* Build friendships. Come across as a person, not as an employee or manager or someone out to get something.

Listen

As you go up in your career, listening to others becomes more and more crucial to your job. The executive must be a sensitive listener, not only for her or his own sake, but because their position of authority affects other people's lives and careers. Be a good listener:

* establish an agreeable and pleasant atmosphere, so that the person you are listening to can feel relaxed
* be prepared to hear the people through on their own terms. Many of the messages worth listening to are not always presented well or in an inviting tone of voice
* be briefed on the subject to be discussed
* avoid getting sidetracked
* listen to even those aspects that you disagree with
* listen for and summarise basic ideas – this is a good device for grasping what is being said and preventing misunderstandings.

People can communicate obliquely. In your organisation learn the language and what it means. Power is often misunderstood.

* 'We're having an impromptu meeting. Come along if you want to.' If you are not at that meeting you may miss something very important.
* 'Don't worry, but ...' means you should worry.
* If you are offered a challenge or an opportunity, you are going to be given a tough job.

The most successful jobholders map out their careers, they do not leave everything to chance. Plan your career so that it fulfils your capacities, needs and dreams.

* What are your dreams? Where do you want to see yourself?
* What are your strengths, your assets, both in the job and out of it?

- What are your weaknesses? What kind of work do you fail in or wish to avoid? What areas do you need to strengthen yourself in? What areas of knowledge or self-cultivation must you pursue?
- What kind of lifestyle do you wish to achieve? What range of income and what kinds of perks?

What will the manager of the future do?

- Plan strategically.
- Organise.
- Motivate, develop and feed back.
- Clarify aims and objectives.
- Measure (formally and informally).
- Self-assess.
- Analyse.
- Respond to and manage change.
- Delegate responsibility.
- Manage:
  - resources
  - people
  - activities
  - information
  - energy
  - quality
  - projects.

For this they will need:

- knowledge
- behavioural skills (assertiveness, communication, influencing skills)
- complex cognitive abilities
- self-knowledge
- emotional resilience
- personal drive.

The motivation to manage

Do you have:

- a favourable attitude towards authority? Rebels never go far in any management hierarchy
- the desire to compete – especially with peers?
- the desire to assert yourself and take charge?
- a desire to exert power and authority over people?

- a desire to behave in a distinctive and different way?
- a desire to take visible and calculated risks?
- a high tolerance for routines, repetitive, detailed paperwork?
- attention to detail?

These components are directly and reliably related to managerial success in terms of productivity, promotions and pay.[3] Cultivate them if you wish to succeed.

References

1 Phillips A (2002) *Communication and the Manager's Job*. Radcliffe Medical Press, Oxford.

2 McGill I and Beaty L (1992) *Action Learning*. Kogan Page, London.

3 Miner J (2000) *The Human Constraint: the coming shortage of managerial talent*. The Bureau of National Affairs, Washington DC.

Further reading

Davidson M and Cooper C (1992) *Shattering the Glass Ceiling: the woman manager*. Paul Chapman Publishing, London.

LaRouche J and Ryan R (1986) Things they never tell you about the office. *Company Magazine*, pp. 32–5. Extract from: *Strategies for Women and Work*. Counterpoint/ Unwin Paperbacks, London.

Martin V and Henderson E (2001) *Managing in Health and Social Care*. Routledge, London.

Mazzei G (1985) Being the boss. *Company Magazine*, p. 75. Extract from: *Moving Up*. Poseidon Press, USA.

Postscript

Having read this book, take some time out to reflect upon how you can put some of the principles into practice. Make a note of your next goal and some of the changes you want to instigate in your life. What action do you need to take to be more assertive? In what situations could you be less aggressive, passive or manipulative? Where do you most need to apply the skills? How will you do it and when?

Having noted what you want to change, work with a friend or colleague to see if your plans are viable, then take charge: sign up to some assertiveness training and begin to make it happen. Those around you – your family, friends and work colleagues – will begin to notice the changes in your conduct. Gradually you will develop your autonomy and allow yourself the freedom to determine your own actions and behaviours. With this will come the confidence and authority to influence those around you more effectively.

Index